Psychotherapy for Bipolar Disorders: An integrative approach

While medication is hugely important in treating bipolar disorders, an integrated approach which utilises psychological treatments can target some aspects that medication alone cannot reach. A comprehensive review of evidence-based psychological treatments is provided, followed by practical information on psychoeducation for patients and family members, healthy lifestyle promotion, mindfulness-based interventions and cognitive and functional remediation, as they represent the basis on which the integrative approach is developed.

The last part of the book provides the sessions of integrative therapy, which can be shared with patients themselves, enhancing the effectiveness of applying the treatment. *Psychotherapy for Bipolar Disorders: An Integrative Approach* offers a brief but multi-component treatment framework that can also be implemented in non-specialised health centres. This approach may greatly improve the well-being and quality of life of people with bipolar disorders.

This accessible text is an essential resource for psychiatrists, clinical psychologists and any healthcare provider working in mental healthcare.

T0201482

Psychotherapy for Bipolar Disorders

An Integrative Approach

Edited by

María Reinares, PhD
Bipolar and Depressive Disorders Unit of the Institute of Neuroscience, Hospital Clinic, IDIBAPS, CIBERSAM, Barcelona, Spain

Anabel Martínez-Arán, PhD
Bipolar and Depressive Disorders Unit of the Institute of Neuroscience, Hospital Clinic, IDIBAPS, CIBERSAM, Barcelona, Spain

Eduard Vieta, MD, PhD
Bipolar and Depressive Disorders Unit of the Institute of Neuroscience, Hospital Clinic, University of Barcelona, IDIBAPS, CIBERSAM, Barcelona, Spain

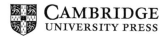

CAMBRIDGE
UNIVERSITY PRESS

CAMBRIDGE
UNIVERSITY PRESS

University Printing House, Cambridge CB2 8BS, United Kingdom

One Liberty Plaza, 20th Floor, New York, NY 10006, USA

477 Williamstown Road, Port Melbourne, VIC 3207, Australia

314–321, 3rd Floor, Plot 3, Splendor Forum, Jasola District Centre,
New Delhi – 110025, India

79 Anson Road, #06–04/06, Singapore 079906

Cambridge University Press is part of the University of Cambridge.

It furthers the University's mission by disseminating knowledge in the pursuit of
education, learning, and research at the highest international levels of excellence.

www.cambridge.org
Information on this title: www.cambridge.org/9781108460095
DOI: 10.1017/9781108589802

First published 2020

Printed and bound in Great Britain by Clays Ltd, Elcograf S.p.A.

A catalogue record for this publication is available from the British Library.

Library of Congress Cataloging-in-Publication Data
Names: Reinares, María, editor. | Martínez-Arán, Anabel, editor. | Vieta, Eduard, editor.
Title: Psychotherapy for bipolar disorders: An integrative approach / edited by María Reinares, Anabel Martínez-Arán, Eduard Vieta.
Description: Cambridge, United Kingdom ; New York, NY : Cambridge University
Press, 2019. | Includes bibliographical references and index.
Identifiers: LCCN 2019015918 (print) | LCCN 2019016847 (ebook) | ISBN 9781108460095 |
ISBN 9781108460095 (pbk. : alk. paper)
Subjects: | MESH: Bipolar Disorder – therapy | Psychotherapy – methods
Classification: LCC RC516 (ebook) | LCC RC516 (print) | NLM WM 171.7 | DDC 616.89/5–dc23
LC record available at https://lccn.loc.gov/2019015918

ISBN 978-1-108-46009-5 Paperback

This study has been funded by Instituto de Salud Carlos III through the project "PI17/00914" (Co- funded by
European Regional Development Fund/European Social Fund) "Investing in your future".

....

Contents

List of Collaborators vii
Preface ix

Part 1 An Introduction to Treatments

1.1 Introduction to Bipolar Disorders 1

1.2 Adjunctive Psychological Treatments in Adults with Bipolar Disorders 6

Part 2 The Foundations of an Integrative Approach to Bipolar Disorders

2.1 Psychoeducation for Patients and Family Members 17
   2.1.1 Distinctive Aspects of Psychoeducation for Patients with Bipolar Disorders 18
   2.1.2 Distinctive Aspects of Family Psychoeducation for Patients with Bipolar Disorders 24
   2.1.3 Psychoeducational Module in the Integrative Approach 30

2.2 Promotion of a Healthy Lifestyle 31
   2.2.1 Characteristics of a Programme Promoting a Healthy Lifestyle in Those with Bipolar Disorder 32
   2.2.2 Promotion of a Healthy Lifestyle Module in the Integrative Approach 39

2.3 Mindfulness 40
   2.3.1 Distinctive Aspects of Mindfulness 41
   2.3.2 Mindfulness Module in the Integrative Approach 49

2.4 Cognitive and Functional Remediation 50
   2.4.1 Distinctive Aspects of Functional Remediation for Patients with Bipolar Disorders 55
   2.4.2 Cognitive and Functional Enhancement Module in the Integrative Approach 60

Part 3 An Integrative Approach to Bipolar Disorders

3.1 Introduction to the Integrative Approach 61

3.2 Contents of the Integrative Approach 64
   3.2.1 Bipolar Disorder: Causes and Triggers 64
   3.2.2 Symptoms of Bipolar Disorder: Early Detection of Warning Signs and Early Action 66
   3.2.3 Treatment of Bipolar Disorder and Therapeutic Adherence 70
   3.2.4 Regularity of Habits and a Healthy Lifestyle 73
   3.2.5 Psychoeducation Directed at Family Members: Family and Bipolar Disorder 82

3.2.6 Mindfulness I: Automatic Pilot versus Awareness 84

3.2.7 Mindfulness II: Habits of the Mind and the Importance of the Body 88

3.2.8 Mindfulness III: Thoughts and Emotions 91

3.2.9 Cognitive and Functional Enhancement: Attention and Memory 94

3.2.10 Cognitive and Functional Enhancement: Executive Functions 101

3.2.11 Problem Solving Skills Training 104

3.2.12 Assertiveness and Communication Skills 106

Appendix 1 The Group Rules 110

Appendix 2 Level of Satisfaction with the Intervention 111

Bibliography 112

Index 120

Collaborators

Brisa Solé, PhD

C. Mar Bonnín, PhD

Èlia Valls, BSc

Esther Jiménez, PhD

Carla Torrent, PhD

José Sánchez-Moreno, BSc

Preface

Pharmacological treatment is essential for the management of bipolar disorder. However, supplementing this treatment with certain psychological treatments has been shown to improve the prognosis of the illness and therefore the well-being of people suffering from it.

The integrative approach proposed in this book is based on the need to cover different areas that may be affected by bipolar disorder, by means of a brief intervention that can therefore be generalised to clinical practice. It intends to include broader therapeutic objectives that make it possible to work on the prevention of relapses without losing sight of other important issues for people suffering from the disease, such as those related to daily functioning, cognition (attention, memory, executive functions), the presence of mild symptoms that often persist between episodes, physical health, well-being and quality of life. To this end, it incorporates therapeutic components of broader psychological approaches that the Barcelona Bipolar and Depressive Disorders Unit developed and whose efficacy has been evaluated separately, such as psychoeducation, family intervention and functional remediation. In addition, it places emphasis on the promotion of a healthy lifestyle and also includes a module of mindfulness-based cognitive therapy. This book is born, therefore, from the authors' clinical practice, teaching and research on bipolar disorder, undertaken over the course of more than two decades and involving patients and relatives as active participants in the therapeutic process.

The book consists of two well-differentiated sections divided into three parts. The first section (Parts 1 and 2) is addressed to mental health professionals. It includes an introduction to bipolar disorder and presents the main efficacy studies in psychological interventions. Then, each of the programmes on which the integrative approach is based is described in detail; this allows the pillars on which this integrative therapy is based to be contextualised. The second section (Part 3), informative and accessible to all types of readers, including those with bipolar disorder and their families and caregivers, presents the contents of each of the 12 sessions of the integrative approach.

Although it has not been easy to select the main components of the different treatments, we are confident that this approach will help guide professionals and reduce the suffering that bipolar disorder generates in patients and families, facilitating strategies to better manage the illness and mitigate its possible consequences. The reality of the disease is too complex to fragment it, hence the importance of an integrative approach that connects different aspects from a biopsychosocial perspective.

Chapter

Introduction to Bipolar Disorders

What Is Bipolar Disorder?

Bipolar disorder, previously known as manic-depressive syndrome, is a chronic and recurrent mental illness that affects the mechanisms that regulate mood and may result in a high level of personal, familial, social and economic burden.

It is estimated that bipolar disorders affect approximately 2.4% of the global population (Merikangas et al. 2011). The illness onset typically occurs during young adulthood, although the diagnosis is often delayed, worsening the long-term prognosis (Altamura et al. 2015). Therefore, an early diagnosis is crucial to establishing an appropriate treatment plan as soon as possible.

To date, the diagnosis of the disease is based on purely clinical criteria. The defining symptoms for mental illnesses are detailed in the *Diagnostic and Statistical Manual of Mental Disorders* (DSM), published by the American Psychiatric Association, and in the International Classification of Diseases (ICD), produced by the World Health Organization. Through psychiatric interviews, clinicians can assess whether the criteria for behaviour changes specific to the disease are met.

Patients with bipolar disorder can show manic, hypomanic and depressive episodes, alternating with symptom-free periods (euthymia). However, some patients complain of persistent residual symptoms (Baldessarini et al. 2010) that, although they do not meet the clinical criteria necessary to be considered a relapse, have a negative impact on cognition (processes such as attention, memory and executive functions which involve planning, organisation and decision making, among other tasks), psychosocial functioning and quality of life (Bonnin et al. 2012; Morton et al. 2018).

Both manic and hypomanic episodes are characterised by a distinct period of abnormally and persistently elevated or irritable mood together with hyperactivity, high energy, increased self-esteem, grandiosity, increased talkativeness, decreased need for sleep, becoming easily distracted, flight of ideas, increased goal-directed activity or psychomotor agitation and excessive involvement in activities that have a high potential for painful consequences (e.g. engaging in unrestrained buying sprees, sexual indiscretions or unwise business investments). Hypomania is less intense than mania and its impact on psychosocial functioning is therefore lower and, in contrast to what can happen in mania or even depression, does not imply psychotic symptoms (delusions and/or hallucinations), nor does it require hospitalisation.

Regarding depressive episodes, a common feature is the presence of lowered mood or a loss of interest or pleasure, together with decreased energy, sadness, feelings of worthlessness or excessive guilt, psychomotor agitation or retardation, decreased ability to think

1

or to concentrate, social withdrawal, insomnia or hypersomnia and low self-esteem. In some cases, recurrent thoughts of death or suicide can appear.

In any phase, some patients can exhibit symptoms at both ends of the spectrum simultaneously (hypomania/mania and depression), known as mixed symptoms.

Depending on the severity and duration of mood episodes, bipolar disorders can be classified as bipolar I disorder (at least one manic episode), bipolar II disorder (hypomanic and depressive episodes), a milder form known as cyclothymia (symptoms of depression and symptoms of hypomania for at least 2 years but not sufficient to fulfil criteria for a major depressive episode or a hypomanic episode) and residual categories of atypical forms that do not fit in the abovementioned subtypes (Vieta et al. 2018).

What Are the Biological Bases of Bipolar Disorder?

Bipolar disorder is a complex disease in terms of both its clinical presentation and its possible causes. Studies indicate that genetic and environmental factors play an important role.

The disease arises as a result of complex interactions involving biological, psychological and social variables. While environmental factors, such as stressful negative events or taking or abusing drugs, can act as triggers for an episode, biological factors, and more specifically genetic predisposition, can be directly related to the cause of the disease.

From a biological perspective, there is consensus that mood disorders are associated with alterations in the limbic system (Figure 1.1). The limbic system is responsible for our mood being regular, stable and appropriate to the environment. Therefore, this brain structure, composed of the thalamus, hypothalamus, amygdala and hippocampus, is responsible for regulating both emotions and some cognitive processes involved in learning capacity and memory.

Of all the neurotransmitters (chemical substances that are responsible for the transmission of signals from one neuron to another), dopamine, serotonin and noradrenaline have been the most studied in relation to bipolar disorder. Alterations of neurotransmission systems play a fundamental role in the different phases of the disease. For example, most

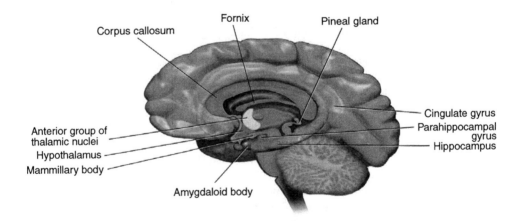

Figure 1.1 Limbic system.

drugs that have been shown to be effective in treating depressive or hypomanic/manic relapses act on this group of neurotransmitters. It is also known that alterations in the release of other neurotransmitters, such as acetylcholine, glutamate and gamma-aminobutyric acid (GABA), could also play an important role.

The neuroendocrine system, responsible for hormonal release, has also been linked to bipolar disorders. The presence of thyroid alterations in a substantial number of patients and the increased risk of suffering a depressive or manic episode after childbirth are some of the factors that reinforce the implication of this system in bipolar disorders.

What Role Does Genetics Play in Bipolar Disorder?

Bipolar disorder does not present a Mendelian inheritance pattern (one gene, one disease) but rather follows a complex pattern of inheritance involving a large number of genes with minor effects whose expression can be modulated by a wide range of environmental factors. It has also been hypothesised that bipolar disorder would respond to what is known as the 'susceptibility threshold model'. According to this inheritance model, the ability to develop this psychiatric condition would follow a continuous distribution among the general population and only those individuals who exceed the threshold would develop it (Mellerup et al. 2012).

Bipolar disorder aggregates in families. Family studies demonstrate that the risk of suffering from bipolar disorder among first degree relatives is approximately 9% (Barnett & Smoller 2009). Furthermore, it is common for relatives of bipolar patients to have an increased risk of unipolar depression and other psychotic disorders such as schizophrenia or schizoaffective disorder.

Twin studies are aimed at determining the weight of genetic variability in the inheritance of bipolar disorder. In this type of study, the concordance rates of monozygotic and heterozygotic twins are compared. Bearing in mind that monozygotic twins share 100% of their genetic information and dizygotic twins only half, results indicate that genetic concordance in bipolar disorder ranges as high as 45% between monozygotic twins and only 5–6% in the latter. Therefore, although genetic variability largely contributes to the total variability of the phenotype, the influence of environmental factors cannot be ignored (Barnett & Smoller 2009).

What Factors Influence the Clinical Course of Bipolar Disorder?

Biological, clinical and psychosocial factors play a significant role in the course and prognosis of the disease.

Although the risk of recurrence may persist even in patients with a good medication adherence, in these cases the frequency, intensity and duration of the episodes are expected to be lower. Unfortunately, a high proportion of patients with bipolar disorder have a poor adherence to their pharmacological treatment, an aspect that undoubtedly has a negative impact on the course of the illness (Levin et al. 2016).

A higher number of previous episodes is related to an impaired quality of life, higher disability and severe persistent symptoms (Magalhaes et al. 2012). These data are especially relevant, as many patients present mild or subsyndromic symptoms (that do not meet acute episode criteria), particularly depressive, between episodes and during long periods (Baldessarini et al. 2010). It has been observed that the shorter the duration of euthymia (stability), the greater the incidence of both residual symptoms and difficulties in daily functioning (Samalin et al. 2016). Therefore, the longer the time without relapses, the better the prognosis becomes. Some studies have reported that a higher number of previous episodes was associated with greater deficits in cognition (Lopez-Jaramillo et al. 2010; Sanchez-Morla et al. 2018) and psychosocial functioning (Rosa et al. 2012), highlighting the relevance of relapse prevention. Psychosocial functioning seems to be directly influenced by both clinical variables (e.g. number of episodes, subsyndromal depressive symptoms) and cognitive deficits (Reinares et al. 2013; Sanchez-Moreno et al. 2018; Sole et al. 2018). Psychosocial functioning and cognitive enhancement have become new targets in the treatment of bipolar disorders, because a high proportion of patients show difficulties outside of the acute phases. In fact, many patients, especially those with a more severe course of the disease, complain of difficulties in attention, memory and executive functions (Martinez-Aran et al. 2004) as well as psychosocial difficulties (Sole et al. 2018) even while in remission.

Stress can act as a trigger of affective relapses (Lex et al. 2017). The social environment in the form of childhood adversities or trauma and stressful life events in adulthood (Gilman et al. 2014), as well as a negative family atmosphere (Reinares et al. 2016), plays a crucial role in the course of bipolar disorder.

The illness is associated with high mortality rates (Hayes et al. 2015) not only because of a high suicide risk (Nordentoft et al. 2011), which can be drastically reduced with an early diagnosis and good treatment, but also because of the high probability of comorbidity, that is, of presenting other psychiatric and/or medical illnesses that often accompany bipolar disorder (Crump et al. 2013). Substance abuse is particularly common in those with bipolar disorders and can negatively affect the course of the illness (Messer et al. 2017). Therefore, there is increasing awareness of the need to promote physical health through the development of regular physical exercise, healthy eating habits and a healthy lifestyle, including the regularity of sleep (which is crucial in bipolar disorder), good stress management and avoidance of substance abuse, all aspects that could also reduce the risk of relapses.

Following other branches of medicine, in which the use of clinical staging has been established (i.e. oncology) to determine the extent and severity of a disease, there have been suggestions that clinical staging could be applied to bipolar disorders, based on emerging data about the potentially deteriorating nature of the illness if not treated early and correctly (Berk et al. 2017). For this reason, early diagnosis and appropriate treatment are of fundamental importance. Clinical staging defines not only the extent of progression of a disorder at a particular point in time, but also the point at which a person is currently on the continuum of the course of a disease. Several staging models have been proposed with the aim of guiding prognosis and helping clinicians to choose the treatment that is better adapted to the patient's needs (Salagre et al. 2018). However, more research is still needed in this area.

What Treatments Are There for Bipolar Disorder?

Pharmacological treatment is essential in bipolar disorders. However, the disease represents one of the psychiatric disorders of greatest therapeutic complexity, because the management of the illness involves the acute treatment of manic, hypomanic and depressive episodes as well as maintenance therapy to prevent future relapses (Grande et al. 2016). Therefore, for any acute intervention, its potential impact on the long range of the illness should be considered. As a metaphor, it could be said that any clinician considering treating a person with bipolar disorder should use 'trifocal' lenses, that is, do not lose sight of near, intermediate and distant vision when selecting the treatment. At the same time, it is important that the pharmacological treatment is well tolerated, with few short- and long-term side effects. Because of the chronic and recurrent nature of bipolar disorder, most experts advocate for a focus on maintenance from the first episode. The choice of maintenance pharmacological treatment will be determined by the patient's clinical history and response to previous treatments.

Following clinical guidelines, mood stabilisers alone or in combination with antipsychotics, or in specific cases with antidepressants, represent the main pharmacological treatment (Goodwin et al. 2016; Yatham et al. 2018). If a manic or depressive predominant polarity can be established throughout the course of the illness (defined as at least twice as many episodes of one pole over the other), it could also contribute to guiding the treatment choice (Popovic et al. 2012).

Psychological interventions also play a crucial role as adjunctive treatment in bipolar disorder, especially when used in patients who are stable or exhibit mild symptoms, as different studies have proved (Reinares et al. 2014). To date, the evidence of psychological approaches in the acute phases of the disease is limited, for obvious reasons in the case of mania but more surprisingly in that of depression. The latter may be due to the tendency, based on an erroneous assumption, to extrapolate the results of unipolar depression (experienced by people who have depression only, without hypomanic or manic episodes) to patients with bipolar depression (depression alternating with episodes of hypomania and/or mania). Although there are areas of overlap between both forms of depression, some differences have also been found: bipolar depression is characterised by earlier age of onset, psychomotor inhibition, higher risk of psychotic symptoms and more atypical depressive symptoms such as excessive sleepiness or increased appetite. The impact of antidepressants is also different, being clear for unipolar patients and unclear and sometimes self-defeating for bipolar patients (Pacchiarotti et al. 2013), increasing the risks of mood shift into hypomania/mania or rapid cycling (the presence of four or more distinct episodes of depression, mania, or hypomania during a 1-year period). Regarding psychotherapy, although a few studies focused on bipolar depression have shown promising findings (Miklowitz et al. 2007), most data about the efficacy of psychological treatments come from samples of patients in euthymia or with mild symptoms. The main evidence-based studies and new approaches are discussed in the next section.

The advantages of combining pharmacological and psychological approaches would contribute to decreasing the burden of bipolar disorder by ensuring the achievement of syndromal recovery from the acute phase and maintaining it through relapse prevention, and also symptomatic and functional recovery, which is crucial for the quality of life and well-being of patients and the people close to them.

Chapter 1.2

Adjunctive Psychological Treatments in Adults with Bipolar Disorders

Why Is It Important to Complement Pharmacological Treatment with Psychological Therapy?

Considering the recurrent and chronic nature of bipolar disorder, optimal long-term management requires a preventive strategy that includes pharmacological treatments together with psychological therapies that have shown efficacy in bipolar disorder. Adjunctive psychological interventions, always as an added treatment to the pharmacological therapy, would ensure the effect of medication through the promotion of adherence to therapy regimen (MacDonald et al. 2016), which is often suboptimal in those with bipolar disorder (Levin et al. 2016), and would address other aspects that medication alone cannot reach.

Different psychological treatments have been developed and tested in bipolar disorder. Although many approaches share some components, the emphasis given to them varies between treatments (Reinares et al. 2014).

The following contains a list of targets of psychological treatments in bipolar disorder:

- ✓ Educating about the illness and its treatment.
- ✓ Correcting myths, false beliefs and misattributions.
- ✓ Replacing self-stigmatisation with acceptance and awareness.
- ✓ Enhancing medication adherence.
- ✓ Stabilising sleep/wake cycles and daily routines.
- ✓ Avoiding substance use.
- ✓ Promoting healthy habits.
- ✓ Improving early detection and treatment of first signs of relapse.
- ✓ Training in stress management.
- ✓ Teaching emotional self-regulation skills.
- ✓ Improving cognitive functioning.
- ✓ Improving psychosocial functioning.
- ✓ Improving well-being and quality of life.
- ✓ Training in social skills to improve interpersonal relationships.
- ✓ Improving family environment, giving support, and promoting self-care, education and skills training for relatives to cope with the illness and manage stress.

Ideally, the needs, characteristics of the subjects and course of the illness should guide the design or selection of the treatment in the context of personalised patient care.

Unfortunately, and despite the recommendation of clinical guidelines (Goodwin et al. 2016; Yatham et al. 2018), some studies report that only a minority of individuals with bipolar disorder receive adjunctive psychotherapy (Barbato et al. 2016; Sylvia et al. 2015).

What Psychological Approaches Have Been Most Commonly Used in Bipolar Disorders and What Scientific Evidence Exists for Them?

The main studies are highlighted here. Most of them are clinical trials (experimental evaluation to assess the efficacy of a given treatment), controlled (the group receiving the treatment under investigation is compared with a group receiving a placebo or a standard treatment such as pharmacological treatment only) and randomised (the research participants are assigned by chance to either the experimental group or the control group).

Cognitive-Behavioural Therapy (CBT)

The cognitive-behavioural therapy (CBT) model focuses on the close relationship between thoughts, emotions and behaviours, and aims at helping the individual to monitor, examine and change dysfunctional thinking and behaviours associated with mood states.

Based on a meta-analysis carried out by Chiang et al. (2017), CBT is effective in decreasing the risk of relapse and improving mood symptoms and psychosocial functioning, with a mild-to-moderate effect. However, the studies as well as the interventions included were highly heterogeneous. When trials have been analysed in greater detail, mixed results have been reported.

Positive findings in terms of number of episodes and days in an episode, admissions, mood symptoms and social functioning were obtained in a 12-month study with 103 bipolar patients randomised to 14 sessions of CBT or a control group (Lam et al. 2003), but at 18 months the effect of CBT in relapse reduction was not significant (Lam et al. 2005). The loss of efficacy throughout the follow-up was also found in other studies (Ball et al. 2006), suggesting the need for booster sessions. Another work reported that the combination of CBT plus brief psychoeducation was superior to brief psychoeducation alone in relation to reducing the number of days in depressed mood (Zaretsky et al. 2008). The long-term efficacy in terms of symptoms and social-occupational functioning of an approach that combined CBT and psychoeducation has also been described (Gonzalez et al. 2012).

No differences were found in a 2-year UK study in which 20 sessions of CBT were compared with support therapy (Meyer & Hautzinger 2012). However, the latter also included certain 'active' components (i.e. information about bipolar disorder and systematic mood monitoring). Similarly, a study headed by Dr Jan Scott (Scott et al. 2006), also in the UK, did not find differences between CBT (22 sessions) compared with treatment as usual in a sample characterised by a highly recurrent course and complex presentations. Interestingly, they found that CBT was effective exclusively in a subgroup of patients with fewer than 12 episodes, suggesting the importance of introducing the treatment as early as possible. In this line of research, a pilot study with individuals with recent-onset bipolar disorder showed that recovery-focused CBT significantly improved personal recovery and increased time to any mood relapse (Jones et al. 2015).

Psychoeducation

Psychoeducation provides education and coping skills training to those suffering from the illness in order to enhance their resources for relapse prevention and empower them to participate actively in the illness management.

One of the first rigorous studies in the area of psychoeducation consisted of 7–12 individual sessions for teaching patients to identify early symptoms and seek prompt treatment. This specific component of psychoeducation proved useful to increase the time to the first manic relapse, social functioning and employment at 18 months; however, the intervention did not prevent depression (Perry et al. 1999). In a group format, the efficacy of adjunctive psychoeducation was shown with a sample of 120 euthymic bipolar patients randomised to receive 21 sessions of group psychoeducation or non-specific group meetings. The psychoeducational programme consisted of five modules focused on illness awareness, the early detection of new episodes, medication adherence, substance abuse avoidance, regular habits and stress management. Psychoeducation reduced the percentage of, number of and time to recurrences and hospitalisations per patient, with benefits observed not only at 2-year follow-up (Colom et al. 2003) but also at five years (Colom et al. 2009) when, together with the long-lasting prophylactic effects, subjects who received psychoeducation had been acutely ill for shorter periods. In addition, the cost efficacy of group psychoeducation was proved by reducing the number of hospitalisations and emergency visits (Scott et al. 2009). However, the clinical benefits of the intervention were especially evident in patients with a lower number of previous episodes (Colom et al. 2010). In a 12-month study with a similar design but shorter treatment length (16 sessions), de Barros et al. (2013) found no differences between groups in mood symptoms, psychosocial functioning and quality of life. The authors suggested that characteristics of the sample could have explained the findings, as patients with a more advanced stage of disease might have a worse response to psychoeducation. Similarly, a multicentre randomised controlled trial conducted at eight community sites in England compared 21 two-hour weekly sessions of either structured group psychoeducation or unstructured peer support for patients with remitted bipolar disorder (Morriss et al. 2016). No differences were found at 96 weeks in terms of patients with new episodes or time to next bipolar episode. However, when the results were analysed in detail, psychoeducation was most beneficial in participants with one to seven previous bipolar episodes, highlighting again the need to provide psychoeducation early in the course of the illness. In Canada, Parikh and collaborators (2012) reported similar clinical improvements when 6 sessions of group psychoeducation were compared with 20 sessions of individual CBT. Using a shorter programme (8 sessions) and including patients with few previous episodes (median of 4), Chen et al. (2018) conducted a study in China that showed the benefits (fewer recurrences in mania in particular, lower rates of rehospitalisation, fewer symptoms and better functioning) of group psychoeducation compared with regular free discussions for inpatients with bipolar I disorder who were in remission from a manic episode.

It is worth mentioning that psychoeducation is also a core element of some approaches involving different components or care packages, some of which have shown positive results on relapse prevention (Castle et al. 2010), manic symptoms (Bauer et al. 2006; Simon et al. 2006), social role function and quality of life (Bauer et al. 2006).

Family Intervention

The illness affects not only patients but also their relatives, who suffer the consequences of the episodes and usually become the main caregivers. Many studies support the negative influence of relatives' highly expressed emotion (presence of criticism, hostility or emotional over-involvement) in the course of the illness. The simultaneous impact of bipolar disorder on family caregivers has also been described, generating a high level of objective burden (alterations in the lives of family members as a result of the illness) and subjective burden (understood as the psychological impact of the illness on family members). This bidirectional relationship should be considered when planning the therapeutic approach (Reinares et al. 2016). Therefore, it is crucial to help the family accept and understand the illness and its treatment, correct false beliefs or attributions, learn strategies to cope with the illness, and reduce stress and negative patterns of interaction.

Several studies support the efficacy of adjunctive family-focused treatment in reducing relapses and increasing time to relapse (Miklowitz et al. 2000; Miklowitz et al. 2003). The treatment, developed by David Miklowitz and colleagues in the USA, consisted of 21 one-hour sessions of psychoeducation, communication enhancement training and problem-solving training delivered at home for the patient and relatives during the post-episode period. The treatment was particularly useful for depressive symptoms (Miklowitz et al. 2003), and was also shown to reduce the hospitalisation risk compared with individual treatment (Rea et al. 2003). In Italy, a multicentre study showed that family psychoeducation delivered to patients and their relatives was beneficial in terms of patients' social functioning, patients' depressive symptoms and relatives' burden (Fiorillo et al. 2014). However, the benefits are not as clear in patients in an acute episode (relapse). Miller and collaborators (2004) reported that neither adjunctive family therapy nor adjunctive multi-family group therapy improved the recovery rate compared with pharmacotherapy alone, except for a subgroup of patients from families with high impairment, in which any modality of family intervention (always added to pharmacological treatment) reduced the number of depressive episodes and time in depression (Miller et al. 2008).

Carer-focused interventions have been shown to diminish family burden (Madigan et al. 2012; Perlick et al. 2010; Reinares et al. 2004). In addition to their positive impact on relatives (Baruch et al. 2018), it seems that even without patients' direct participation there are benefits in relapse prevention, as a network meta-analysis recently concluded (Chatterton et al. 2017). In a 15-month randomised controlled trial carried out in Barcelona, twelve 90-minute group sessions of psychoeducation delivered to caregivers of euthymic adults with bipolar disorder reduced the risk of recurrence and delayed the emergence of new recurrences, particularly (hypo)mania, in comparison with treatment as usual (Reinares et al. 2008). The contents of this programme will be detailed in Part 2. Other authors have shown the benefits on patients' affective symptoms and carers' health risk behaviour, subjective burden and depressive symptoms of a family-focused, health-promoting intervention (Perlick et al. 2010; Perlick et al. 2018).

Interpersonal and Social Rhythm Therapy (IPSRT)

Interpersonal and social rhythm therapy (IPSRT) is based on the hypothesis that stressful life events and unstable or disrupted daily routines can lead to circadian rhythm instability and, in vulnerable individuals, to affective episodes. Circadian rhythm refers to the inherent cycle of about 24 hours that appears to control various biological processes, such as sleep and wakefulness.

One of the main studies on IPSRT was conducted by Dr Ellen Frank and collaborators (2005) at the University of Pittsburgh and involved 175 acutely bipolar patients, 2-year follow-up and four treatment options, depending on the treatment (IPSRT or intensive clinical management consisting of education) to which each patient was assigned in the acute and maintenance phases. No differences were found in terms of time to remission, nor in the proportion of patients achieving remission. However, patients who received IPSRT in the acute treatment phase survived longer without an episode and showed higher regularity of social rhythms. Regularity during acute treatment was associated with a reduced likelihood of recurrence during the maintenance phase. Subjects who initially received IPSRT showed more rapid improvement in occupational functioning but no differences at the end of the follow-up (Frank et al. 2008). Similarly, more rapid improvement of mood symptoms but a comparable response rate were found by Swartz et al. (2017) in a study of patients with bipolar II disorder in a depressive episode randomly assigned to 20 individual sessions of IPSRT plus quetiapine (to a maximum of 300 mg/day) or IPSRT plus placebo in identical-appearing capsules. IPSRT plus quetiapine assignment was associated with a significantly higher body mass index over time and rates of a dry mouth. Patients randomly assigned to their preferred treatment were 4.5 times more likely to respond. Finally, Inder and others (2015) randomised a group of 100 participants with bipolar disorder to IPSRT or specialist supportive care. After treatment, both groups had improved depressive symptoms, social functioning and manic symptoms. The reduction in symptoms was maintained at 3-year follow-up for both conditions (Inder et al. 2017).

Are There New Approaches to Bipolar Disorder?

Cognitive and Functional Remediation

A close connection between cognitive deficits and poorer psychosocial functioning has consistently been reported (Sanchez-Moreno et al. 2018). In bipolar disorder, cognitive deficits in attention, memory and executive functions have been described not only during acute phases but also in euthymia (Martinez-Aran et al. 2004), with a high level of variability and heterogeneity in subgroups of patients with a similar profile in terms of cognition (Burdick et al. 2014; Sole et al. 2016) or psychosocial functioning (Reinares et al. 2013; Sole et al. 2018). Therefore, treating cognitive impairment has become an important therapeutic target (Miskowiak et al. 2018). Through different strategies the treatment aims to improve cognitive performance and daily functioning.

A group from the University of Copenhagen (Demant et al. 2015) carried out a randomised controlled trial with bipolar patients in partial remission and with cognitive complaints assigned to 12 weeks of group-based cognitive remediation or standard treatment. Cognitive remediation had no effect on cognitive or psychosocial functioning. The authors suggested that longer-term, more intensive and individualised cognitive remediation may be necessary to improve cognition. In contrast, positive results were obtained by Lewandowski and colleagues (2017) with an Internet-based cognitive remediation programme (70 hours) in comparison with a dose-matched computer control. At post-treatment, better performance was obtained in processing speed, visual learning and memory, and the cognitive composite score; superior processing speed and cognitive composite was maintained 6 months after the intervention. Cognitive remediation was not associated with a change in community functioning.

Functional remediation consists of an intervention involving neurocognitive techniques and training and education in cognition and problem solving within an ecological framework, with the main aim of improving functional outcomes in bipolar disorder. In Spain, Torrent and other authors (2013) carried out a randomised trial that involved several centres, with a total of 239 euthymic patients with functional impairment. The sample was divided into three subgroups according to treatment: 21 sessions of group functional remediation, 21 sessions of group psychoeducation, or treatment as usual. The functional remediation programme resulted in improving patients' psychosocial functioning, but no significant effect of treatment group on the clinical (manic and depressive symptoms) or neurocognitive variables was found at the end of the intervention (6 months). However, at 1-year follow-up, the benefits of functioning were maintained and an improvement in verbal memory was obtained (Bonnin et al. 2016). This approach represents a useful option for the high proportion of patients with problems of poor functioning.

Mindfulness-Based Cognitive Therapy (MBCT)

At the core of mindfulness-based interventions is the ability to keep one's attention focused non-judgementally in the present moment (Kabat-Zinn 1994). It involves an attitude of acceptance to help one to observe rather than react to thoughts, emotions and bodily sensations and to respond more skilfully.

Mindfulness-based stress reduction (MBSR) (Kabat-Zinn 1990) and mindfulness-based cognitive therapy (MBCT) (Segal et al. 2001) are the main mindfulness-based interventions. Both share the same format and structure (eight weekly sessions of 2 hours each) but MBCT replaces some of the content of MBSR with a focus on specific patterns of negative thinking to which people with depression are vulnerable. Mindfulness has also been incorporated as part of other treatment modalities such as dialectical-behavioural therapy or acceptance and commitment therapy.

In contrast with other areas, little research has been conducted on mindfulness-based interventions in subjects with bipolar disorder. In the few controlled studies that included bipolar patients using MBCT, a reduction in anxiety and depressive symptoms (Williams et al. 2008) and an improvement in emotional regulation (Ives-Deliperi et al. 2013) have been reported. Similarly, a decrease in anxiety scores for bipolar patients allocated to MBCT compared with treatment as usual was found in a trial with 95 patients followed over 12 months (Perich et al. 2013a). However, no differences were observed between groups in depressive or manic symptoms, time to recurrence and number of recurrences. When the impact of mindfulness practice was examined, a significant correlation was found between a greater number of days spent meditating during the 8-week MBCT programme and lower depression scores at the end of follow-up (Perich et al. 2013b), stressing the importance of practice. Recent reviews reported the benefits of mindfulness on anxiety and depressive symptoms, cognitive functioning and emotional regulation in bipolar disorder (Bojic & Becerra 2017; Lovas & Schuman-Olivier 2018), although a meta-analysis (Chu et al. 2018) suggested that most positive results derived from uncontrolled trials, highlighting the need for further rigorous research with this population in this field.

Internet-Supported Psychological Interventions

There is increasing access to the Internet in the general population, and therefore several programmes using the Internet have been developed for patients with bipolar disorder, as has been comprehensively described in recent reviews (Faurholt-Jepsen et al. 2018; Gliddon et al. 2017; Hidalgo-Mazzei et al. 2015). Internet-based interventions can be divided into two broad categories according to their main platform of delivery: web-based interventions (e.g. ORBIT, MoodSwings, Beating Bipolar, Bipolar Education Program, Recovery Road, Living with Bipolar, iCBT, MoodChart, MyRecoveryPlan) and mobile-based interventions (e.g. MONARCA, PRISM, SIMPLe). Most of the evidence concerning bipolar disorders comes from web-based programmes which, however, do not provide objective monitoring but are aimed more at delivering interventions and remotely monitoring symptoms. In mobile technology, there is the possibility of continuously capturing objective behavioural data and complementing self-reported measures, while at the same time delivering interventions outside clinical settings. Finally, even though these platforms are appealing, they share challenging issues such as retention and engagement, suggesting they should use a feasible and acceptable method of delivery. As in face-to-face psychological treatments, future studies should clarify which components of the programmes are crucial in relation to obtaining expected results. Another issue is finding a balance between the degree of patient self-management and the level of clinician involvement. Many studies are at a preliminary stage, making it difficult at present to draw firm conclusions about the effectiveness of psychological interventions using Internet-supported technologies for bipolar disorders. Meanwhile, we cannot dismiss their utility as a complement of current treatments.

Recently, through the combination of objective measures (actigraphy and ecological momentary assessment) and subjective measures through the traditional clinical method, Merikangas and collaborators (2018) observed a close relationship between parameters such as motor activity, energy, mood and sleep hours. The findings suggest the importance of active and passive tracking of multiple regulatory systems and the need to integrate all these aspects in order to achieve a more effective therapeutic approach.

Other Approaches in a Preliminary Phase of Study

The adaptation of different therapeutic approaches to the field of bipolar disorders has begun to be studied. The following summarises some of them:

Dialectical Behaviour Therapy (DBT). DBT may be an effective adjunct treatment for improving emotion regulation and residual mood symptoms in patients with bipolar disorder. This approach works towards helping subjects increase their emotional and cognitive regulation by learning about the triggers that lead to reactive states and helping to assess which coping skills to apply to avoid undesired reactions. Preliminary studies using DBT with bipolar patients have been conducted, with positive results seen in depressive symptomatology and emotional control (Goldstein et al. 2015; Van et al. 2013).

Eye Movement Desensitisation and Reprocessing (EMDR). EMDR uses a standardised eight-phase protocol which involves making side-to-side eye movements or other bilateral stimulation, while simultaneously focusing on symptoms and experiences related to the traumatic event, incorporating elements of cognitive, interpersonal and body-centred therapies. The application of this therapy to bipolar disorders is based on the negative impact of traumatic events on a more severe course of the illness over time (Aas et al. 2016). A promising preliminary study has been done (Novo et al. 2014), and a multicentre study is under way (Moreno-Alcazar et al. 2017), the results of which may better define the role this therapy can play in bipolar disorder.

Metacognitive Training. This method was first developed to improve metacognitive abilities in patients with schizophrenia (Moritz & Woodward 2007). An open pilot study in bipolar disorder highlighted the feasibility and utility of the intervention using psychosocial functioning as a main outcome, but the lack of a control group means it is not yet possible to draw conclusions about its efficacy (Haffner et al. 2018).

Lifestyle Interventions. Although maintaining a healthy lifestyle is important in bipolar disorder and is usually a component of different approaches, research on diet and exercise has recently begun, and treatments particularly aiming at improving healthy habits are still scarce in this population (Bauer et al. 2016). Most randomised controlled trials have been carried out with mixed samples of patients with severe mental illness, including unipolar depression, schizophrenia and bipolar disorder (De Rosa et al. 2017). One randomised controlled trial conducted in a sample of patients with bipolar disorder used a 20-week cognitive-behavioural intervention consisting of three modules: nutrition, exercise and wellness (Sylvia et al. 2013). Over the course of the treatment, participants showed improvements in exercise, nutritional habits, depressive symptoms and overall functioning. Previously, with a 5-month intervention of 11 group sessions and weekly fitness training, another randomised controlled trial reported a reduction in body mass index, particularly in female patients (Gillhoff et al. 2010). A positive impact on weight loss was found in a behavioural intervention in a mixed sample that also included bipolar patients (Daumit et al. 2013). Results from open trials of exercise as an adjunctive intervention for bipolar disorder have reported that more physical exercise means fewer depressive symptoms, better quality of life and increased functioning, as well as less psychiatric comorbidity (Melo et al. 2016).

Bipolar disorder is a chronic mental illness with dramatic changes in mood. The illness leads to a high level of personal, familial, social and economic burdens. As previously stated, although medication is essential in bipolar disorder, in the past two decades there has been a growing interest in the development of adjunctive psychological interventions in order to enhance aspects that medication alone cannot reach and to account for the heterogeneity of areas of intervention.

As was reviewed in the section on evidence-based adjunctive psychological treatments, the efficacy of specific psychological interventions has been proven not only in short- but also long-term follow-up for some treatments; many interventions share components, but vary in the emphasis given to them (Reinares et al. 2014). The main outcomes also differ, with most psychological treatments focusing on the prevention of episodes of mood swings. Recently, however, the importance of improving other areas affected by the disease, such as cognition, psychosocial functioning, physical health, persistent symptoms, well-being and quality of life, is being underlined.

The duration of the therapies, usually approximately 20 sessions, is an important aspect to consider, especially for many psychological treatments that have been shown to be effective: group psychoeducation of patients, some family intervention programmes (e.g. family-focused treatment), cognitive-behavioural therapy, interpersonal and social rhythm therapy, and functional remediation. It is necessary to generalise intervention programmes developed in specialised centres to the usual clinical practice. This requires the design and evaluation of potentially effective treatments that must be brief and feasible enough to be implemented more widely. In the same way, making the inclusion criteria more flexible would make it possible to cover a greater number of patients and would be more representative of the population with bipolar disorder.

An integrative intervention is therefore required that combines the main components of different approaches to cover broader therapeutic objectives, to improve the prognosis of the disease in both clinical and functional aspects, as well as the well-being and quality of life of those who suffer from the illness. Because of its characteristics and its potential lower cost, this intervention could be easily applicable to routine clinical practice.

The integrative approach incorporates therapeutic components of other broader treatments that the Barcelona Bipolar and Depressive Disorders Unit has developed and whose effectiveness has been evaluated separately, such as psychoeducation, family intervention and functional rehabilitation. In addition, an important emphasis is given to the promotion of a healthy lifestyle, and a module focused on mindfulness-based cognitive therapy is included.

This section, Part 2, describes the treatments previously mentioned that represent the foundation on which the development of the integrative approach is based. In Part 3, the contents of each of the 12 sessions of the brief integrative approach are outlined and discussed.

Psychoeducation for Patients and Family Members

Every illness represents in some way a threat and increases the sense of vulnerability. The diagnosis of a chronic and recurrent mental disorder influences a person's self-image and has a strong impact on all members of the family. In the adjustment to the diagnosis, each individual usually undergoes a process in which a variety of beliefs and emotions may arise that will have to be dealt with, in parallel to education about and acceptance of the disorder. It is common for denial to appear first, attributing what has happened to external factors. There is also a tendency for the patient to deny the chronic nature of the disorder, refusing the possibility that another episode may occur. The onset of the disease can often be accompanied by a marked sense of loss, experienced both by the person receiving the diagnosis and by his or her relatives: the loss of the healthy self together with an increase in the feeling of vulnerability, real losses as a consequence of the episodes (work is impaired, social difficulties arise, ruptures occur, family are affected, financial problems ensue, etc.) or perceived loss, sometimes erroneously, of expectations about the person him- or herself or about the future. There may be a tendency for the person to define her- or himself by the disorder ('I am bipolar') rather than being able to distinguish between illness and identity ('I have a bipolar disorder') which goes far beyond any diagnosis. Added to this, there is the marked stigma that still surrounds mental illness and that leads many people to hide the disorder even from those in their closest circles for fear of rejection or embarrassment. Statements such as, 'People with bipolar disorder are violent and unpredictable', 'Bipolar disorder is always disabling', 'Individuals with bipolar disorder have a double personality' are unfortunately very common. They reflect the myths and ignorance that still exist about mental illness, and as such should be reviewed and corrected. All these aspects of reactions to diagnosis are potentially modifiable and should therefore be considered in the therapeutic approach and throughout whatever may be required in the process of acceptance of bipolar disorder.

In medical illnesses such as diabetes, asthma or high blood pressure, the need for education about the factors that can improve the course of illness seems self-evident. The same should be true for mental disorders. The knowledge and acceptance of bipolar disorder, as well as the optimisation of strategies for its management, will not only contribute to increasing the sense of control and self-efficacy but will also positively influence the course of the disorder, which is the primary goal of any treatment. Although all types of interventions with some educational component are often erroneously included within the psychoeducational approach, a distinction must be made between merely transmitting general information and those treatments that incorporate theoretical and practical skills training in order to allow the subjects to take an active role in the therapeutic process.

Psychoeducation can have a crucial impact on both disease awareness and therapeutic adherence, and consequently on the prognosis of bipolar disorder. In addition, aspects such as early detection of warning signs and other factors such as maintaining healthy and regular habits and managing stress are essential pillars for the prevention of relapses, as different studies discussed previously have shown. Therefore, it is essential that patients and their families receive support, education about the disease and training in coping strategies that have a positive impact on the course of the disorder and consequently improve their well-being and quality of life.

Several psychoeducation manuals have been developed for clinicians working with patients with bipolar disorder (Bauer & McBride 2003; Colom & Vieta 2006) or with the family, the latter in different formats such as family-focused treatment directed at the whole family unit (Miklowitz & Goldstein 2007) or caregiver-focused psychoeducation (Reinares et al. 2015).

Two psychoeducation programmes, one for patients and one for relatives, are presented in the following sections. Both have inspired the psychoeducational module of the integrative approach presented in Part 3 of this book.

2.1.1 Distinctive Aspects of Psychoeducation for Patients with Bipolar Disorders

What Is Psychoeducation?

Psychoeducation is a therapeutic approach that attempts to provide a theoretical and practical framework in which those who suffer from the illness can better understand and face the disorder and its possible consequences, actively participating in treatment (Table 2.1). It replaces the model of a 'healing' professional and a 'passive' patient with that of an appropriate therapeutic alliance based on collaboration, information and trust (Colom & Vieta 2006).

Psychoeducation goes beyond the mere transmission of information. Psychoeducation leads to cognitive and behavioural changes, for which it must involve training in practical skills that improve the subject's competence in coping with the disease. It is based on the medical model and highlights the relationship between vulnerability and environmental factors that can act as triggers or protectors of relapses during the course of the disorder.

How and When Should Psychoeducation Be Implemented?

Psychoeducation can be carried out in an individual or group format. Working with groups is not only a less expensive option but also offers a very appropriate framework for working on disease awareness and fighting stigma. In addition, groups facilitate modelling or

Table 2.1 Distinctive aspects of psychoeducation

Psychoeducation involves replacing …
– Mere information → education and training in coping strategies
– Illness denial → awareness and acceptance of the illness
– Guilt → responsibility
– Helplessness, passivity → proactive attitude
– Hierarchical therapeutic relationship → therapeutic relationships relying on information, collaboration in decision making and trust
– Inflexible appointment system → easy accessibility to clinicians and on-call availability
– One clinician → multidisciplinary team

observational learning and increase the support and social network of participants. It is advisable to work with a co-therapist and to include approximately 10 patients per group. The group can form in a semicircle around the therapists, promoting interaction and communication, which can include a black- or whiteboard. It is important to use the time well to ensure that in each session doubts are resolved and the planned contents are covered, promoting dialogue and discussion. The use of exercises and the formulation of questions will encourage the participation of all attendees.

The process of learning about the disease should begin the moment it is diagnosed and from that point constantly expanded, allowing the patient's and the therapist's understandings to be in alignment. However, psychoeducational intervention as a specific treatment, as will be discussed later, has been implemented in a group format and tested in subjects who were on medication and whose mood was stabilised at the time of the intervention. This makes it possible to highlight a fundamental objective of the treatment: the prevention of relapses.

What Are the Components of the Psychoeducational Programme for Patients with Bipolar Disorder?

In Section 1.2 on the efficacy of psychological treatments in bipolar disorder, different studies on psychoeducation and its level of scientific evidence were described. As mentioned, one of the main studies was carried out by Colom and collaborators to evaluate the efficacy of group psychoeducation with a sample of 120 euthymic bipolar patients who were followed for 2 (Colom et al. 2003) and 5 years (Colom et al. 2009), with very positive results in relapse prevention. To date, this programme represents, owing to its characteristics and the studies carried out, one of the most recognised in psychoeducation. Proof of this is the fact that psychoeducation, always as a complement to medication, is part of the therapeutic recommendations for the treatment of bipolar disorder in the maintenance phase, according to noted clinical practice guidelines for the management of bipolar disorder (Goodwin et al. 2016; Yatham et al. 2018).

The programme consists of 21 group sessions of 90 minutes each (Figure 2.1), structured in five blocks and whose contents and implementation have been described in greater detail in a manual by Colom and Vieta (2006). After each session, previously prepared material summarising its contents is distributed.

What follows is a brief description of the content of the five modules that make up the programme, in addition to a few practical exercises to consolidate aspects related to the modules on awareness of the illness and early detection of mood episodes.

1. Awareness of the Disorder

Within the framework of the stress–vulnerability model, the disease manifests as a result of the interaction between vulnerability (or genetic predisposition) and environmental factors that may precipitate its onset or influence the evolution of the disorder. The biological, chronic and recurrent nature of bipolar disorder is then highlighted. Working on these aspects is crucial for understanding and accepting the need for long-term treatment. In this context, establishing the distinction between causes (emphasising the biological basis of the disease) and triggers (or environmental factors that can influence relapses) is made clear. It also places the person in an active and responsible position by realising that, although the risk of relapse is always present, certain behaviours can reduce such risk and contribute to keeping the disease under control. Therefore, awareness of bipolar disorder will enhance protective

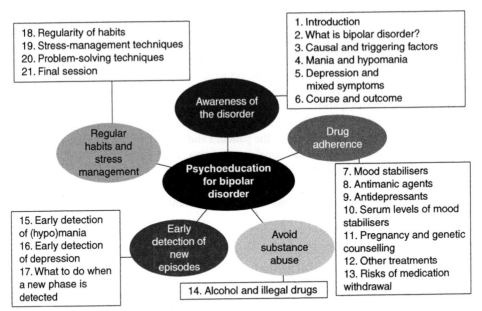

Figure 2.1 Sessions of the group psychoeducational programme for bipolar disorders (Barcelona Bipolar and Depressive Disorders Unit).

factors that will ensure a better prognosis, such as good adherence to medication, avoidance of drug abuse, regularity of habits and stress management. An issue that may interfere with the acceptance of the disease has to do with social stigma and shame, often built on myths and erroneous beliefs that must be identified and corrected from the first session. Working with groups provides an ideal environment for destigmatisation. Symptoms specific to each episode are reviewed in this module, highlighting the (often underestimated) pathological character of hypomania and aspects related to the course of the illness.

A useful exercise for this block of sessions consists of drawing a graph with the evolution of the illness during the past approximately 8–10 years. On a horizontal line reflecting the state of euthymia over time, the different types of episodes experienced are represented (with elevations for hypomania, more accentuated elevations for mania and reductions illustrating depressions) as shown in Figure 2.2. At the same time, it is helpful to write down the dates corresponding to the relapses, possible triggers (if there were any), the consequences of the episodes and the treatment received.

This exercise allows the subject to detect specific patterns (e.g. if there is a seasonal pattern – coinciding with certain seasons of the year – or if the relapses have occurred after potential triggers such as drug use), as well as to be more aware of the chronic and recurrent nature of bipolar disorder, and not to underestimate the risks associated with relapses (hospitalisations, breakups, socio-occupational problems, overspending, etc.).

2. Drug Adherence

Pharmacological treatment is essential for bipolar disorder, and its abandonment or poor adherence is a clear predictor of relapses, with all the complications that these entail (hospitalisations, cognitive deficits, problems with work and social functioning, increased risk of suicide, etc.). The fact that almost all people who suffer from bipolar disorder have

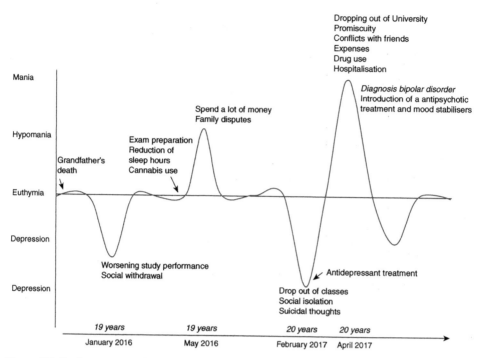

Figure 2.2 Graph representing the course of the illness.

thought, throughout their lives, of abandoning the treatment, and that approximately half of them have done so on some occasion – even in periods of euthymia – justifies the importance of having sessions on adherence. The patients are informed about the different pharmacological treatments for the disorder and their therapeutic and adverse effects. Doubts and fears are addressed and erroneous beliefs about the treatment corrected (i.e. 'People with bipolar disorder lack lithium in their blood', 'Pharmacological treatment creates addiction', 'Medication prevents experiencing emotions', 'Memory problems are exclusively caused by pharmacological treatment'). Identifying the factors that influenced poor adherence in the past, and what the consequences of poor adherence were, can help prevent it from happening again. Explaining the phases that a drug goes through before being introduced to the market and familiarising patients with the scientific method generates greater confidence. It can also be useful to later state which non-pharmacological approaches have – and which have not – shown efficacy in bipolar disorder. In this module, medication and other recommendations related to pregnancy are also addressed, always highlighting the importance of advance planning and psychiatric counselling.

3. Avoiding Substance Abuse

This aspect takes on an important role because of the high level of correlation between bipolar disorder and substance abuse or dependence, as well as the fact that the latter may act as a trigger for relapses and is a predictor of a more unfavourable course of the illness. Drug abuse or dependence is usually an exclusion criterion in many studies on the efficacy of pharmacological and psychological treatments. Therefore, even if the group's patients do not have serious drug abuse problems, it is important that any programme with bipolar patients highlights the need to avoid certain types of substances. Many bipolar patients engage in sporadic or non-abusive drug use that can cause negative effects. Cannabis, which many patients do not qualify as a harmful drug, should not be overlooked, and it is therefore advisable to explain all its dangerous effects. Along with illegal substances, which patients are recommended to avoid completely, the negative effects of alcohol should be discussed. Instructions should also be given regarding the consumption of caffeinated beverages such as coffee or other stimulant drinks. These should be avoided in the afternoon and evening because of their potential negative impact on sleep (which can act as a trigger for relapses), and eliminated altogether in the case of hypomanic/manic symptoms and episodes.

4. Early Detection of New Episodes

Early detection of the first warning signs (called prodromes) of new episodes is an essential ingredient of psychoeducation and a very useful strategy to teach those with bipolar disorder. The development of an individualised prodrome list, following the guidelines discussed here, can be a useful tool for calibrating behaviour and for early detection of the onset of relapses. The compilation of such a list requires exhaustive work that consists of transforming the initial lists drawn up by the patient, often constituted by symptoms (i.e. 'I sleep 4 hours') or non-specific indicators (i.e. 'I sleep less'), into alarm signals that imply **qualitative** or **quantitative** changes as objectively as possible.

A helpful exercise consists of drawing up a list of about 10 prodromes for hypomania/mania and 10 for depression. To make the list as operative as possible, a valid prodrome should be based on the following:

- Observable **behaviour**, because emotions are more subjective and difficult to evaluate. The behaviour is **objectively measurable** and easily identifiable.
- **Subtle** signs, because otherwise it would count as a symptom. The focus is on early detection, so for that reason it is better to choose warning signs that could potentially escalate to symptoms.
- Presence on a **regular** basis before the previous episodes.
- Being evaluable **daily**.
- Involving a certain **distinction** from the person's temperament and habits.

Table 2.2 reflects some examples of the process of creating the list of operational warning signs. The aim is to convert non-specific statements into more concrete prodromes. The limits established in the quantitative or qualitative changes will always depend on the temperament, usual functioning and routines of the person when stable.

Once the list has been created with the help of the therapist, the patient should review it daily and, if he or she identifies the presence of three or more prodromes, activate an 'emergency plan' that includes contacting the psychiatrist among other measures of taking prompt action. The psychoeducational programme also provides precise guidelines to be followed when warning signs of hypomania or depression are identified.

5. Regular Habits and Stress Management

Regularity of habits and stress management play an important role in reducing the risk of relapses in bipolar disorder, which is the reason both factors should be included in any psychoeducational programme. This module emphasises the need to maintain a healthy lifestyle that incorporates regular physical exercise and an adequate eating pattern, as well as

Table 2.2 Creation of a list of prodromes

Non-specific	Concrete
'I sleep less'→	'I wake up before the alarm clock rings'
	'I sleep fewer than 7 hours'
'I eat less'→	'I skip meals'
'I am more active'→	'I go to the gym every day'
	'I am incapable of sitting around watching a movie'
'I feel more spiritual'→	'I started going to church'
	'I started to read books on spirituality'
'I smoke more'→	'I smoke more than 15 cigarettes a day' (or another figure that represents some increase from the usual average)
	'I started smoking joints'
'I change my style of dress'→	'I wear miniskirts and brightly coloured clothes'
	'I wear sleeveless shirts and a hat'
'I underestimate the risks'→	'I drive faster than I am allowed'
	'I have unprotected sex'
'I am more sociable'→	'I talk to strangers'
	'I dedicate more than (number) hours to social networks on the Internet'
'I am more irritable'→	'I argue with my partner'
	'My family tells me I am more irritable'

an average of 8 hours of sleep as a protective factor and strategies for stress management such as relaxation and problem-solving training. These aspects will be further developed in the sections on promoting a healthy lifestyle and mindfulness.

Is It Possible to Control Mood and Learn about Bipolar Disorder via Mobile Phone?

Despite their effectiveness, psychoeducational treatments are not always available in all centres and are not adapted to the schedules and locations of all who need them. Conversely, in recent years mobile devices connected to the Internet have become a common tool in the lives of a large part of the population. More and more people are turning to the Internet for information about their illness and strategies for better management of it. These factors have contributed to the recent development of various devices intended to be a tool for better mood management, as discussed in Part 1.

The aforementioned aspects have led to the development of a mobile application that incorporates the contents of the psychoeducational programme previously presented with the aim of studying the usefulness of mobile devices in monitoring patients diagnosed with bipolar disorder. Self-Monitoring and Psychoeducation in Bipolar Patients with a Smartphone application, or SIMPLe, facilitates the constant recording of mood, while providing personalised psychoeducational messages aimed at contributing to maintaining mood stability. Everything is presented in a simple, friendly and discreet way to ensure the minimum possible interference and maximum compliance with absolute confidentiality. The user can customise the best time of the day to answer the test questions and receive the psychoeducational messages at his or her convenience.

The application is based on the idea that every day the person will answer test questions about mood state, hours of sleep, energy level, irritability and medication taken. After doing so, he or she receives a personalised psychoeducational message. In the event that the answers to the daily test detect warning signs, a more exhaustive test is activated, which is otherwise systematically presented on a weekly basis. If a risk of decompensation is suspected, the patient is advised to contact his or her doctor of reference or go to the emergency services. Simultaneously, the application allows users to do things such as programme warnings at established times for taking medication, to incorporate information on prodromal symptoms of relapse in order for the device to warn of its possible appearance, to record stressful events and to share the mood graph with other people. Regular use of the application is reinforced by medals and trophies as a way of boosting motivation.

The application is continuously being tested to scientifically evaluate its efficacy and safety (https://simplebipolarproject.org/). To date, it has shown high levels of feasibility, adherence – especially in the first months – and satisfaction (Hidalgo-Mazzei et al. 2016, 2018) as well as having a positive impact on adherence to medication and circadian rhythms (Hidalgo-Mazzei et al. 2017). Translations from Spanish to other languages are currently under way, which will allow this resource to be offered more widely to users. Work is also being done to complement the subjective data, introduced by the person with the disorder, with objective data (sleep, activity level, Internet browsing, etc.) captured through mobile phones or through smartbands.

Through the use of smartphones, other applications such as MONARCA (MONitoring, treAtment and pRediCtion of bipolAr disorder episodes) (Faurholt-Jepsen et al. 2014, 2015) and PRISM (Personalized Real-time Intervention for Stabilising Mood) (Depp et al. 2015) have also been developed for those with bipolar disorder.

The integrative approach proposed in Part 3 of this book provides patients with information on SIMPLe and other applications, as well as links related to the contents of the programme with the aim of reinforcing each module worked on during the intervention.

2.1.2 Distinctive Aspects of Family Psychoeducation for Patients with Bipolar Disorders

Why Is It Important to Involve Family Members?

Bipolar disorder affects not only the patient but also the people with whom he or she lives. Bipolar disorder and family functioning affect each other.

On the one hand, each episode of the illness represents a stressful event for all members of the family and generates painful emotions, worry and disturbance of the family balance. It also involves changes in established roles and requires the development of coping strategies specific to the crisis situation. It is common for family members to ignore their own needs and, even in periods of stability during the illness, fear of future episodes often persists, which can be a source of constant anxiety. Therefore, the illness and its consequences can affect the daily functioning of family caregivers, as well as their physical and mental health, especially if they do not receive the support, information and training they need. This objective and subjective impact of the illness on caregivers has been called 'family burden'.

DENIAL	HYPERVIGILANCE
Poor therapeutic adherence	
Failing to encourage recommended behaviour	
Attribute symptomatic behaviours to the patient's will	
Unrealistic expectations	
Criticism	
Anger	
Conflicts	
	Overprotection
	Difficulties setting limits
	Limiting patient's aspirations and autonomy for fear of relapses
	Interpreting any behaviour or emotion as pathological
	Over-identification with the caregiver role, disregarding other roles and neglecting their own needs and those of other members
	Co-dependency
	Anxiety

Figure 2.3 Emotional reactions and their consequences.

On the other hand, the family can influence the level of stress both positively and negatively, becoming the best ally or the main obstacle to effective treatment (Reinares et al. 2015). Studies on expressed emotion have shown that the presence of relatives' critical comments (e.g. 'She does not collaborate in housework'), hostility (e.g. 'He is lazy') and/or emotional over-involvement (e.g. 'I am constantly looking out for her; if she is not nearby, I cannot relax') has a negative influence on the course of the illness. However, the clinician must be cautious in the way this information is transmitted to relatives and avoid any kind of blaming but still emphasise a reality: the relationship between the person with the illness and the family is reciprocal. Family psychoeducation aims to reinforce favourable attitudes and, in the case of group intervention, to take advantage of this context to model and encourage behaviours that may reduce the level of stress and improve the family atmosphere.

Not only the person diagnosed with bipolar disorder but also the family members may find it difficult to accept and understand the nature of the disease. A continuum could be established whose extremes are at one end denial and at the other hypervigilance (Reinares et al. 2015). Each of these attitudes elicits consequences that could affect the course of the illness (Figure 2.3). Sometimes different members of the family may adopt different positions (e.g. a father who denies the illness and a mother who adopts an overprotective attitude) and this also becomes a source of conflict to be addressed. A whole range of emotions can be placed along the continuum, such as frustration, a feeling of loss, sadness, fear for the future, anxiety and guilt, among others. Some family members have also reported positive aspects of their role as caregivers, such as the enhancement of feelings of love, pride and compassion.

Given the close relationship between attributions, attitudes and behaviours, it is impor-tant to identify and work on the beliefs that different members of the family may have about the illness in order to correct them in a way that leads to more beneficial behaviours for themselves, the family environment and the course of the disorder. Carer emotional reactions and behaviours will be completely different depending on their appraisals. For example, it has been observed that if a family member is highly critical, there may be a tendency to attribute symptoms and certain behaviours to factors controllable by the patient, whereas underlying overprotection may be a tendency to attribute the behaviour to factors beyond the patient's control (Lobban et al. 2003). The aim is to use emotions constructively and encourage changes to positions that are more beneficial for the patient and the family members themselves, facilitating acceptance and a proactive attitude through the use of adaptive coping strategies that also increase a sense of control and self-efficacy.

In summary, the impact of a stressful family environment – characterised by the family's attitudes/behaviours such as a highly expressed emotion and a negative affective style – on the course of the illness, the burden experienced by those who live with the patient (which can affect their own daily functioning as well as their physical and mental health), and the family's demand for more information about bipolar disorder and their coping strategies are some of the reasons to support the introduction of psychoeducational family interventions for bipolar patients (Reinares et al. 2016).

What Is Family Psychoeducation?

Family psychoeducation involves giving support to the relatives of the patient, encouraging self-care, educating them about bipolar disorder, and training them in coping and stress management strategies, usually through training in communication skills and problem solving.

It is expected that the course of the illness will be more favourable if the family understands and accepts the disorder, controls the factors that can trigger relapses, learns to identify the first signs of new episodes and act accordingly, incorporates skills to manage family conflicts and stress situations appropriately, and adopts attitudes and behaviours that facilitate the management of the illness, such as promoting regularity of habits and adherence to treatment.

How and When Is Family Intervention Delivered?

Family intervention can be administered in different formats: single family unit including the patient, multifamily groups, groups of relatives, and patient and caregiver groups in parallel (Table 2.3).

One negative aspect of the caregiver group concept is that it makes it difficult to address more intimate issues. However, this limitation is overcome if an atmosphere of trust and acceptance is created in which the therapist openly and naturally raises all issues related to the disease. In addition, the possible anxiety that can be generated in some cases by the group format tends to dissipate quickly after the first sessions. However, in the event that highly conflictive family dynamics are detected, an approach aimed at the entire family unit including the patient may be more appropriate. Although in this section we will focus on psychoeducation aimed exclusively at relatives of patients with bipolar disorder, it is in no way intended to replace the individual approach to the person suffering from the illness, but rather to complement it. Ideally, patients and relatives could benefit from parallel psychoeducation groups or from an intervention that integrates patient and caregivers. Studies have shown that both family-focused treatments (Fiorillo et al. 2014; Miklowitz et al. 2003) and carer-focused interventions (Reinares et al., 2008; Perlick et al., 2018) benefit the course of the illness.

Table 2.3 Advantages of different intervention formats

Single family unit	Group of caregivers
✓ A joint intervention involving all parties allows different views to be contemplated. ✓ Observe (and work on) the interaction between the different members. ✓ More personalised approach and objectives. ✓ Work on more intimate aspects that they perhaps do not want to reveal in a group. ✓ It may prevent the relatives of recently diagnosed patients from being alarmed by cases of greater severity. ✓ Resource for those who do not want to attend a group. ✓ More flexible schedule.	✓ Allows the identification and exchange of experiences among equals. ✓ Facilitates expression, normalisation and handling of emotions, without fear of offending the patient. ✓ Allows the modelling of more adaptive coping strategies. ✓ Increases the variety of solutions to problems. ✓ Increases support, social networks and the importance of self-care. ✓ Increases acceptance, illness awareness and destigmatisation. ✓ More economical.

As pointed out in the section on scientific evidence, most family intervention studies have been conducted with patients who were euthymic or with mild symptoms; the results are less consistent when the intervention is introduced in the acute phase (for a more exhaustive review of the subject, see Reinares et al. 2016). One of the advantages of carrying out the intervention when the person is stable is that doing so promotes a climate of less emotional intensity that facilitates the assimilation of information and the resolution of problems. At the same time, it allows the longitudinal perspective in the management of bipolar disorder to be emphasised, highlighting the importance of prevention. Otherwise, there is a risk of focusing the intervention on the search for immediate solutions derived from the period of crisis or of it becoming a resource for emotional venting.

What Are the Components of the Psychoeducational Programme for Relatives of Patients with Bipolar Disorder?

As discussed, there are different formats and types of family interventions. Here we will describe the contents of the psychoeducational programme delivered to family caregivers of patients with bipolar disorder carried out at Hospital Clínic in Barcelona. The patients whose relatives attended the group were in euthymia. The intervention consisted of 12 group sessions of 90 minutes each held once a week (Figure 2.4); the content of the programme has been detailed in Reinares et al. (2015). The programme is similar to the one presented in Figure 2.1 on psychoeducation for patients, but shorter and with greater emphasis on the role of family members, promoting attitudes and behaviours favourable to themselves, for the illness, and also for stress management such as communication skills training.

The integrative approach which is presented in Part 3 of this book includes a session delivered to family caregivers that is based on our experience with the programme as outlined here.

1. Understanding the Nature of the Illness

As a first approach to the illness, the meaning of the disorder for family members is explored. It is worth considering what the illness has represented in their lives, to identify

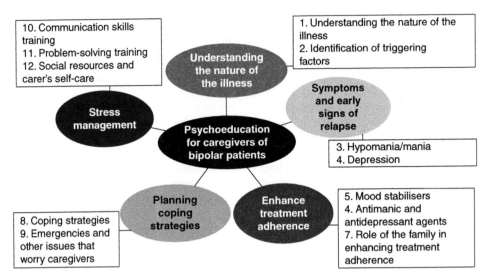

Figure 2.4 Sessions of the group psychoeducational programme delivered to family caregivers of patients with bipolar disorder (Barcelona Bipolar Depressive Disorders Unit).

prejudices about the disorder and its treatment, and gradually correct myths and false beliefs, while enhancing positions that contribute to improving the prognosis. It is essential that the family understand not only the biological, chronic and recurrent nature of the disorder, but also the role that certain environmental factors play in the course of the illness. Therefore, the biological vulnerability to future episodes is highlighted together with the potential negative impact on the illness of triggering factors such as poor pharmacological adherence, drug abuse, unhealthy lifestyle/irregular habits and stress. It is encouraging for family members to know that, despite the chronicity of the disease, certain attitudes and behaviours can reduce the risk of relapse. The role of the family in relation to bipolar disorder is underlined, always from a constructive point of view. Family caregivers often become experts; their experience complemented with the knowledge and training we can offer should improve management of the illness. The feelings of guilt expressed by some relatives have to be dealt with, as well as attitudes of denial, criticism, overprotection or hypervigilance that can lead to conflicts and affect the illness as well as every member of the family. The idea is to help relatives understand and accept the illness.

2. Symptoms and Early Signs of Relapse

It is interesting to encourage the family members themselves to list the characteristic symptoms of each type of episode. From there, a crucial aspect of the intervention focuses on the detection of the first warning signs, both in the face of hypomania/mania and in the face of depression. Family members are often the first to become aware of the onset of new episodes and such recognition, provided it is done in an appropriate manner, will contribute to early intervention and consequently to a better course of the disease. The development of a list of prodromes, as discussed in the section on psychoeducation directed at the patient, may be useful. Adding to the list at home together with the patient can be much more enriching, as well as ensuring a more exhaustive compilation to be revised by the therapist afterwards. Having this tool can reassure family members and help avoid the tendency to interpret any emotional reaction in isolation as pathological.

3. Enhance Treatment Adherence

The family can play a crucial role in therapeutic adherence. Sometimes certain comments guided by prejudice, ignorance, false beliefs or carelessness can have a negative impact on the patient's attitudes and behaviour towards medication. Phrases such as, 'With this medication you look like a zombie' or 'This makes you fat' are just a few examples of comments that can be totally counterproductive. Many family members have concerns, doubts and fears regarding medication and the patient's need for long-term treatment. Underestimating the risk of relapse or the consequences of relapse and overestimating the drawbacks of medication can have a negative impact on adherence. Therefore, it is important to help family members understand the reason for a maintenance pharmacological treatment, identify the associated fears and correct erroneous beliefs about the therapeutic and adverse effects of the medication, as well as encouraging attitudes and behaviours that contribute to enhancing and reinforcing good therapeutic adherence. Care must be taken that medication does not become a source of family conflict. With regard to the role of the family in relation to medication, it is advisable to avoid excessive control (which in any case should be limited to acute phases) and to modify the level of involvement depending on the phase of the illness, promoting the patient's maximum autonomy and responsibility for the medication if the mood is stable.

4. Planning Coping Strategies

Family members should adjust coping strategies according to the different phases of the illness. Strategies that can be useful in the acute phase can be completely counterproductive in euthymia. This requires high levels of flexibility on the part of family members. It is important that expectations are realistic and adjusted to the phase of the illness. Coping strategies will differ depending on whether the person is experiencing the first symptoms of relapse or is in an acute phase, after hospitalisation, or during euthymia (Figure 2.5).

This module should also address emergency situations such as the presence of suicidal ideation or hospitalisation, as well as other issues of concern to the family such as pregnancy, genetic risk, and where to establish the boundary between bipolar illness and personality.

5. Stress Management

Stress management skills training plays a key role in working with families, especially concerning the association between stress and risk of relapses. For this reason, most

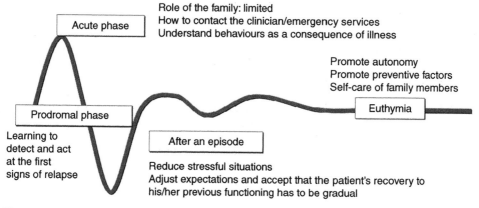

Figure 2.5 The need to adapt strategies and positions according to each phase of the illness.

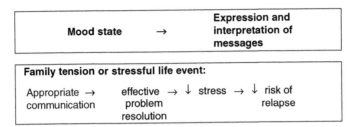

Figure 2.6 Communication and bipolar disorder.

familyinterventions have training sessions in communication skills and problem-solving training.

Communication represents an instrument to link the person suffering from the illness and those around him or her. It is important for the family to understand that mood fluctuations are linked to cognitive changes and have a clear impact on communication, affecting the interpretation and expression of messages (Figure 2.6). For example, the feelings of worthlessness characteristic of depression or the suspicion that sometimes accompanies mania can distort the interpretation of the messages received and affect the way in which the person expresses him- or herself. Therefore, it is essential that the family be aware of the patient's mood at the time of interaction. In the same way, the emotional state of the patient's relatives can influence communication. On the other hand, in the face of a stressful situation or family tension, the type of communication will influence more or less effective problem solving and, consequently, will increase or reduce the level of stress that can act as a trigger for relapses (Figure 2.6).

Not only conflict but also the systematic avoidance of it denote difficulties. The objective is not to avoid topics that are considered important but to know how to select the moment and the most appropriate way to approach them with assertiveness. Reciprocity is the basis of communication and implies that the parties involved are equally responsible for the way in which the interaction takes place. Role-playing is used to work on communication skills training.

As in communication, the patient's symptomatology can also interfere with the resolution of problems. For this reason, it is advisable not to take important decisions in the presence of symptomatology and to postpone them to moments of euthymia, which will favour objectivity and freedom in decision making. When problems implicate other people, the best solutions are those that require an action plan involving the different parties, and this is especially applicable to the family context. Problem-solving training will contribute to finding more effective alternatives.

In the last session of this programme, information is given on the available social and health resources. Finally, the importance of carers' self-care is highlighted, an aspect that has been emphasised throughout the programme, fostering attitudes, behaviours and strategies that have a positive impact on both their health and their quality of life.

2.1.3 Psychoeducational Module in the Integrative Approach

The programmes mentioned previously offer a framework to contextualise part of the contents included in the psychoeducational module of the integrative approach that is presented in Part 3, which also includes a session for relatives. The contents have been selected on the basis of our 20 years' experience of conducting psychoeducation groups, also taking into account feedback from the participants. Information on healthy and regular habits is included and subsequently expanded in the section on promoting a healthy lifestyle.

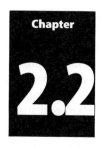

Promotion of a Healthy Lifestyle

What we do throughout life contributes to accelerating or to slowing down the ageing process. Although we tend to remember the importance of taking care of ourselves when we feel ill, good health should be considered a long-term investment. A sedentary lifestyle, obesity, tobacco, consumption of alcohol and other substances, and stress, among others, are factors that negatively affect our cells, accelerating the deterioration of tissues in our body. Good health means staying active physically, intellectually and socially, as well as carrying out healthy and regular habits, including a balanced diet and varied physical exercise. Fortunately, control of these factors is in our hands. If we manage to transform healthy behaviours into habits, the effort to maintain them will be less and will be rewarded by the motivation and perceived benefits for health and quality of life.

Disability-adjusted life years (DALY) is a measure of global disease burden, expressed as the number of years lost due to illness, disability or premature death. It was developed in the 1990s as a measure to compare the overall health and life expectancy of different countries. Bipolar disorder is one of the mental illnesses that generates the highest level of burden (Murray et al. 2012). People with severe mental disorders have mortality rates two times higher than that of the general population; in bipolar disorder, life expectancy is 9 years lower than the rest of the population (Crump et al. 2013). In addition, people living with bipolar disorder present more risk of obesity, hyperglycaemia and metabolic syndrome, all related to risk factors such as lack of physical exercise, unbalanced diet, consumption/abuse of tobacco and alcohol that could be modified through changes in lifestyle.

Low levels of physical exercise have been associated with poorer quality of life, worse overall functioning and more depressive symptoms. In contrast, regular exercise improves cardiorespiratory function and reduces the risk of premature death, in addition to having a positive impact on weight control and cholesterol levels. However, a recent study reported that approximately half of people with mental disorders did not meet the recommendation of at least 150 minutes of physical activity per week, with subjects with bipolar disorder being more likely to have a sedentary lifestyle (Vancampfort et al. 2017). Some of the barriers identified have to do with illness and medication. In terms of eating habits, many people with the disease tend to eat a large amount of saturated fatty acids and large amounts of sugar (simple carbohydrates). This food consumption pattern is associated with diseases such as type II diabetes, dyslipidaemia, obesity, hypertension and cardiovascular diseases. Beyond the genetic predisposition, most of the behaviours associated with these diseases are modifiable (sedentary lifestyle, inadequate nutrition, smoking, etc.) through the implementation of good dietary habits. Diets high in fruits, vegetables, fish and whole grains are associated with a decreased risk of depression (Lai et al. 2014). A study in patients diagnosed with bipolar disorder found that obesity was linked to a worsened course of the disease (Fagiolini et al. 2003).

Helping patients persist with small changes can lead to substantial positive impacts over time; to get to that point, however, it is important that the person accepts that change is needed, finds the motivation to change and overcomes obstacles in the way of making change (Nierenberg et al. 2015). There are few randomised clinical trials studying the efficacy of interventions based on healthy lifestyles exclusively in the bipolar population. Sylvia and collaborators (2013) pointed out the benefits of a cognitive-behavioural intervention consisting of three modules: nutrition, exercise and well-being. After the treatment, participants showed improvement in exercise, nutritional habits, depressive symptoms and overall functioning. Previously, another study had proved the efficacy of an intervention on healthy lifestyle, nutrition and physical exercise on muscle mass index. It was found that women with bipolar disorder improved body composition after receiving this intervention (Gillhoff et al. 2010).

In recent years, health professionals have become increasingly interested in motivating their patients to adopt healthy lifestyles, becoming more physically active and eating a balanced diet as a strategy to prevent disability and improve quality of life. In addition, in bipolar disorder, negative life events and stress may trigger relapses (Lex et al. 2017). Conversely, use of drugs negatively affects the course of the disease (Messer et al. 2017; Starzer et al. 2018). Therefore, regular healthy habits (sleeping an average of 8 hours, eating a healthy diet, avoiding abuse of drugs), controlling the level of stress and being active physically, intellectually and socially are basic ingredients for good health. Hence, the factors explained in what follows will be of fundamental importance for people suffering from this disease. Assuming the responsibility of controlling these factors can reduce the risks and improve the prognosis of the illness, in addition to increasing physical–psychological well-being and quality of life. For this reason, the integrative approach dedicates a session to promoting healthy lifestyles, which is presented in Part 3.

2.2.1 Characteristics of a Programme Promoting a Healthy Lifestyle in Those with Bipolar Disorder

Is There a Recipe for a Healthy Lifestyle?

A key step to implementing a healthy lifestyle involves routine assessments of the state of the disease, as well as developing a baseline state of the target behaviour to change/enhance. It is advisable to act when the person is euthymic or exhibits mild symptoms of the disease. The goal should be working on the motivation for change; otherwise, the possibilities for success are significantly reduced. On the other hand, it is not advisable to try to modify more than one aspect at a time. The idea is to introduce small changes in the daily routine that can be maintained and consolidated over time.

What Ingredients Should the Programme Include?

1. Regularity of Biological Rhythms: The Importance of the Sleep Pattern

Generally, lack of sleep can cause irritability; fatigue; drowsiness; loss of concentration; forgetfulness; reduction of performance and productivity; alteration in endocrine, metabolic and immune systems; reduction of alertness; and an increased risk of accidents.

In bipolar disorder, reduction in sleeping hours may trigger an episode of hypomania or mania. For example, spending a sleepless night or sleeping a few hours could precipitate an episode of euphoria. At the same time, sleep disturbance is a clear symptom in depression as well as in hypomanic/manic episodes. For example, during episodes of mania the person not only tends to reduce the hours of sleep but also has the perception that he or she does not need to sleep, which in turn worsens the clinical outcome. As for bipolar depression, it is often accompanied by excessive sleepiness (hypersomnia). Therefore, in bipolar disorder, sleep can be used not only as a symptom to be treated during a relapse but also as a prevention strategy before a relapse occurs. Thus, a good way to stop the onset of a hypomanic/manic decompensation is to ensure a good number of hours of sleep for several days, while hypersomnia or daytime sleepiness, typical of some depressive episodes, can be managed by reducing the hours of sleep and increasing daily activities. Sometimes, the use of medication may be necessary to improve the sleep pattern, always, however, under medical supervision.

Stress can also affect sleep patterns; it is important to learn to prioritise tasks and manage time adequately, as well as learning training strategies to better cope with stress levels, as will be discussed later in more detail.

The number of sleep hours is crucial in preventing relapses (in bipolar disorder it should fluctuate around 8 hours per day, respecting a fixed schedule for sleep); just as important is the quality of sleep. 'Quality of sleep' refers to sleeping without interruption, allowing 'the batteries to be charged' for good performance during the next day. Therefore, jobs involving night or rotating shifts are discouraged. Changes resulting from trips to areas in different time zones should also be considered, in order to minimise the impact on sleep patterns. Keeping a record of the hours of sleep or using devices (e.g. smartbands) to control it can be a very useful guide to assess biological rhythms and to guide possible interventions if variations are observed. In any case, this should be discussed with the healthcare team.

The specific recommendations for bipolar disorder can be reinforced by **some sleep hygiene guidelines** that are listed in the material on the session corresponding to healthy habits included in the integrative approach presented in Part 3.

2. Dietary Habits

Eating properly is essential for good health. The body needs certain substances (nutrients) to create and maintain the tissues and to get the energy needed to perform vital functions. A healthy diet should be balanced, varied and sufficient, taking into account the characteristics and lifestyle of the individual. A healthy diet provides the necessary amounts of energy and nutrients and minimises the risk of diseases associated with unbalanced consumption, in addition to contributing to the delay in the ageing process.

Variety, balance and moderation in the quantity consumed are basic principles contributing to healthy eating, and this helps maintain body weight. Taste preferences and dietary habits have a lot to do with our learned behaviours. In recent years, eating styles in developed countries have changed considerably, promoting the consumption of fats, sugars and animal proteins and a lower consumption of fibre. A sedentary lifestyle together with poor dietary habits can lead to an imbalance between calories consumed and calories spent, promoting overweight and obesity because of the excessive accumulation of body fat. Besides the physical limitations and the impact of obesity on body image and self-esteem, other important consequences are derived from increasing weight, including an increased risk of cardiovascular disease, diabetes, musculoskeletal disorders,

Table 2.4 Foods for a healthy diet

Increase	Include	Limit
Fruits (avoid juices). Fresh vegetables (green leafy vegetables). Healthy fats (olive oil, avocado, dark chocolate – not less than 85%). Natural or roasted nuts (not fried or salted). Whitefish, bluefish and seafood.	Legumes and vegetable proteins (tofu, soya, green peas). White meat (poultry). Whole grains (bread, flour, rice, quinoa, pasta).	Precooked meals. Red meat. Battered and deep-fried foods. Baked goods and pastries. Butter and hard cheese. Sugary/carbonated drinks. Salt.

Table 2.5 Ways to improve environmental control and conscious eating

Environmental control	Conscious eating
Confine eating to a single space in the house. Plan meals in advance. This can even be done for the whole week. Go shopping on a full stomach. Prepare food when you are not hungry to avoid snacking. Do not buy unhealthy and high-calorie food (pastries, savoury snacks, precooked dishes).	Sit at the table when eating. Eat slowly and in small bites. One strategy is to leave the cutlery on the table every time you take a bite. Devote a few minutes to reflect on the food in the dish (its preparation, cooking, how it is grown). Eliminate distractions during the meal (TV, tablets, mobile phones) and pay attention to the sensations (level of appetite, taste, smells, colours, texture), being aware of the associated emotions and thoughts. Be alert to body signals and stop eating when you feel full.

hypertension, dyslipidaemia, dyspnoea, sleep apnoea, gallbladder disease and some cancers. Obesity, therefore, increases the risk of premature death. One of the most commonly used parameters to measure obesity is the **body mass index** (BMI) that is calculated by dividing the weight in kilograms of the person by their height in metres squared (kg/m^2). According to the World Health Organization, a normal BMI in adults is between 18.5 and 24.9, a BMI of over 25 corresponds to overweight and one above 30 indicates obesity.

It is never too late to promote a healthier diet; however, it is best to establish new habits when the patient is euthymic. Referral to a specialist should be considered if the goal is weight loss or to treat hypertension, diabetes or other endocrine problems. However, if there is motivation to improve eating habits, the following tips may be useful. The ideal diet pattern is similar to the traditional Mediterranean diet which is characterised, among other aspects, by a high consumption of cereals, fruits, vegetables, nuts, legumes and olive oil (as the main source of fat); a moderate consumption of fish, chicken and dairy products; and a low consumption of red meat. Regular consumption of water is also important, because it maintains body temperature and is essential for metabolic functions and the elimination of toxins.

Besides following the recommendations in Table 2.4, the advice in Table 2.5 can be also applied.

Table 2.6 Bipolar disorder medication weight gain risks

High	Moderate	Minimal	Neutral	Low
Clozapine	Lithium	Aripiprazole	Agomelatine	Topiramate
Olanzapine	Gabapentin	Amisulpride	Bupropion	Zonisamide
Chlorpromazine	Mirtazapine	Asenapine	Carbamazepine	
	Risperidone	Haloperidol	Cariprazine	
	Paliperidone	Fluphenazine	Esketamine	
	Pregabalin	SSRI	Lamotrigine	
	Quetiapine	SRNI	Lurasidone	
	Valproate		Oxcarbazepine	
			Vortioxetine	
			Ziprasidone	

SSRI: selective serotonin reuptake inhibitors; SNRI: serotonin norepinephrine reuptake inhibitors

Overeating can be sometimes triggered by emotions. When this happens, eating is used as a tool to reduce anxiety by consuming high-calorie, sugary and fatty foods. 'Emotional hunger' implies that the person eats because of the emotions rather than real hunger. It is important to identify and address this. Some examples include eating when stressed (at work, at school), eating as a response to emotions (sadness, anger, anxiety, boredom, feelings of loneliness or emptiness) or to improve mood (using the food as a crutch), eating with the feeling of loss of control, and even continuing eating despite feeling full. Eating with full consciousness helps to pinpoint why emotional eating is occurring when it does. Treating emotional hunger is important in identifying the triggers that cause it, and to break the relationship established between the triggers and the food intake, which could end up in binge eating.

In the case of bipolar disorder, changes in mood may also involve alterations in appetite that affect the usual eating pattern. Frequently, hyperactivity, common in hypo-manic/manic episodes, leads to skipping meals and depression is accompanied by a reduced intake of food, with the consequent loss of weight, or by excessive intake (hyperphagia). The latter is a characteristic trait in atypical depressions. This, together with the potential effect on weight gain of some pharmacological agents for illness management (Table 2.6), reinforces the importance of promoting healthy habits in this population. In addition, if any unhealthy behavioural pattern is detected, an appropriate referral should be made for treatment. It is also important to explore fears about weight gain or possible side effects of the medication in order to agree on the most appropriate treatment and establish guidelines that limit, as far as possible, the adverse effects of the medication.

The following should be considered in relation to bipolar disorder: (a) follow a healthy and regular food pattern, avoiding excessively restrictive diets that generate hunger and may increase levels of anxiety; (b) there are no 'prohibited' foods, unless antidepressants (monoamine oxidase inhibitors (MAOIs)) are prescribed, in which case the appropriate diet for these medications should be followed; (c) if lithium is prescribed, a low-sodium or sodium-free diet should not be abruptly initiated because it could interfere with lithium blood levels.

A group of scientists from the University of Barcelona validated the Barcelona Bipolar Disorders Eating Scale (Torrent et al. 2008). It consists of a brief, hetero-applied (administered by the clinician) instrument, whose 10 items revolve around the regularity of eating habits, the influence of mood over eating, bingeing behaviour, mechanisms regulating satiety, the tendency to eat compulsively and a craving for carbohydrates. It allows a quick and effective evaluation of the intensity and frequency of eating dysfunctions, guiding clinicians on those aspects that require more attention.

3. Active Lifestyle and Physical Exercise

Being physically active is the ideal complement to a healthy diet. The diet must provide the necessary nutrients and energy to obtain a good energy balance between intake and the energy expenditure required by day-to-day activities.

Physical activity has a positive effect both physically and psychologically, increasing the feeling of well-being. Both an active lifestyle and structured exercise provide numerous health benefits. To ensure consistency over time, it will be better to select exercises that generate some motivation and perform them at least three days a week, combining cardio-vascular exercise with muscle strengthening.

Physical exercise:

- Increases body temperature, producing a relaxing effect.
- Reduces muscle tension.
- Encourages the release of endogenous opioids.
- Reduces depressive symptoms and improves mood.
- Allows for weight control.

Anyone can change his or her lifestyle at any age to become physically active. Nevertheless, it is always advisable to talk with the doctor before starting any physical activity. The best point at which to implement an active lifestyle is during euthymia. The prescription of physical exercise should be personalised, according to the state of health, previous conditioning and motivation. Whatever the person's age and physical condition, there will always be options to stay physically active (Table 2.7).

Some tips for maintaining an active lifestyle:

- Identify physical exercises/activities that the person already performs daily and encourage an increase in the time dedicated to them.
- Combine structured exercise with an active lifestyle in everyday activities (e.g. using the stairs instead of using the lift (elevator)).
- Enhance the social aspects of physical activity as they can contribute to continuing the effort.
- Reinforce patience, persistence and perseverance.

However, there are some considerations to keep in mind regarding exercise and bipolar disorder:

- Because physical exercise is stimulating, it should not be done at night or in the late afternoon, as it could worsen the quality of sleep or cause difficulties in falling asleep.
- In light of a possible episode of mania or hypomania, physical activity should be drastically reduced because it is stimulating.

– Physical exercise can be a very powerful tool during depressive phases. It is helpful to determine which activities are positive for the patient, because they can serve as a resource to modulate mood and increase feelings of well-being.

Table 2.7 Physical activities for positive health effects

Structured exercise	Active lifestyle
Brisk walking to increase heart rate. Strength exercises, such as weight training, squats. Aerobic exercises: running, cycling, swimming, attending gym classes. Activities such as yoga, tai-chi or dance.	Walk to work or to the store instead of going by car or motorcycle. Climb the stairs instead of using the lift (elevator). Park the car farther from the destination. Get off the underground or bus a couple of stops before the final destination.

4.   Avoid Substance Abuse

When talking about promoting good health, it is essential to discuss the importance of avoiding drug abuse. We talk about 'comorbidity' when an individual presents more than one diagnosis simultaneously, and we use the term 'dual pathology' when there is an addictive disorder together with another mental disorder. It is known that the prevalence of addictions is very high in patients living with bipolar disorder. To explain this high association, several hypotheses have been proposed, including self-medication, common vulnerability factors and substance abuse as a risk factor. What we know with certainty is that the abuse of drugs in bipolar disorder adversely affects the course of the disease, increasing the risk of hospitalisations, reducing the response to treatment and worsening the disease prognosis (Messer et al. 2017). In addition, drug abuse impacts the therapeutic approach, because both conditions should be treated simultaneously. Furthermore, sporadic consumption can also trigger a relapse, negatively affecting disease prognosis. There are also people whose substance abuse is restricted to the context of the episodes, which further worsens the clinical outcome.

The effects of illegal drugs (e.g. cannabis, cocaine, hallucinogens or other designer drugs) may act as a trigger that starts a new affective and/or psychotic episode, in addition to promoting behaviours characterised by greater disinhibition, anxiety, impulsivity and even aggressiveness. However, legal substances such as alcohol are also extremely harmful in bipolar disorder. Alcohol is a central nervous system depressant; it increases anxiety and the risk of depression, interferes in sleep patterns, reduces impulse control, causes cognitive impairment and increases aggressiveness. All these substances (legal and illegal) worsen the course of the disease, as discussed in more detail in the session corresponding to this topic presented in Part 3.

Finally, stimulant substances such as caffeine can interfere with the hours of sleep and thus influence the course of the illness. Therefore, it is best to curtail or cease the consumption of coffee, tea and the so-called energy drinks (Red Bull, Monster, etc.) starting early in the afternoon, and eliminate them totally if hypomanic or manic symptoms are present. As for tobacco, it does not directly affect the course of bipolar disorder. However, because of its harmful effect on health, it is best to stop smoking, which should be done during euthymia and under medical supervision to control the increase in anxiety or irritability usually associated with tobacco withdrawal. In addition, some drugs used for detoxification (e.g. bupropion or varenicline) can affect the course of bipolar disorder, and therefore it is better to use nicotine gum or patches.

Misuse of benzodiazepines (anxiolytics and hypnotics) can occur. As inappropriate use of benzodiazepines can lead to dependency, it is important to be careful and always use this medication under medical prescription and supervision.

5. Enhance Well-Being and Coping with Stress

Managing stress is an important part of the process. Lazarus and Folkman (1984) define stress as a particular relationship between the individual and the environment that is appraised by the person as exceeding his or her resources and endangering his or her well-being.

Stress shortens telomeres (the ends of chromosomes) and promotes inflammation, in addition to being associated with unhealthy behaviours. Stress can be a trigger for relapse in bipolar disorder, either directly, through the biological changes it generates, or indirectly, affecting the sleep pattern (which could trigger an episode). For these reasons, stress management should be an essential component of the treatment of bipolar disorder.

There are different types of stressors, from intense one-off life events, through daily stressful events of lower intensity, to situations of chronic sustained tension. Although there is a tendency to associate stressful situations with negative events (e.g. a death, dismissal, breakdown of a relationship), there are positive situations that can also be stressful (e.g. job promotion, marriage). In bipolar disorder, it has been seen that the sign of the episode (mania, depression) does not necessarily correspond with the type of stressor (positive, negative). However, stress is not always harmful; in fact, it helps to maximise the energy resources of the body to survive a threatening situation. Therefore, relatively mild, brief stress that remains under control can be stimulating and even improve a person's performance. However, when it is too intense or maintained over time it leads to the release of cortisol, producing a significant decrease in the immune response which could increase the body's vulnerability to certain infections and diseases. The General Adaptation Model (Selye 1950) suggests that in a stressful situation there is an alarm phase (increasing activation and mobilising defences against the demand), a resistance phase (adaptation to the stressor; if the threat does not disappear there is a gradual distribution of resources by activating the hypothalamic–pituitary–adrenal axis) and, finally, the exhaustion phase, in which the adverse consequences are maintained for longer than the person can withstand them.

Other factors that influence the perception of stress have to do with the novelty of the situation, lack of predictability, uncertainty, situations in which the person does not know what to do or the belief that his or her own resources are exceeded. Coping with stress refers to the strategies developed by the individual with the aim of managing specific external and internal demands assessed as overwhelming or exceeding his or her resources. Various factors can act as modulators of the level of stress: social support, behavioural habits, personal or constitutional variables, coping style (e.g. confrontation using direct actions to alter the situation, distancing in an attempt to forget the problem, self-control with the objective of regulating one's feelings and actions, the acceptance of responsibility, the search for social support, avoidance, positive re-evaluation giving a constructive meaning to the situation in order to deal with it), among others. Therefore, coping styles can vary depending on the stressor and the person.

In the response to stress, cognitive, physiological, emotional and behavioural factors intervene.

The cognitive component (thoughts and beliefs) is a fundamental aspect to consider. It is often not the external demands but the way of perceiving them, that is, the way of interpreting the situation and the assessment a person makes of his or her capacity to face the demands, which in turn determines emotions and reactions. Therefore, being aware of negative automatic thoughts (dichotomous thinking, catastrophism, jumping to conclusions, selective attention ignoring other aspects of the event, etc.) and being able to question them and look for more realistic and evidence-based alternatives, can place someone in another position in the same situation.

At the behavioural level, training in assertiveness, communication skills and problem solving can contribute to a greater perception of self-efficacy in certain potentially stressful situations. In the same way, good planning, prioritisation and time management can facilitate the resolution of the demands that may arise, without forgetting to incorporate rewarding moments and rest into an agenda, as well as enhancing the social life that is a fundamental aspect for well-being.

There are also several strategies that contribute to reducing physiological activation or muscle tension associated with stress. Among the best known are controlled diaphragmatic breathing and Jacobson's progressive muscular relaxation training.

Sometimes, the strategy is more directed at improving emotional regulation than at changing the focus of the situation or the resolution of the problem. In parallel, poor regulation of emotion can interfere in the resolution of problems, as it can lead to impulsive responses. Being less reactive to certain thoughts, emotions and physical sensations puts the situation in a more favourable light. In this context, mindfulness training, defined as deliberately paying attention, in the present moment and without judging, to how the experience unfolds from moment to moment, is important (Kabat-Zinn 1994). This approach will be discussed in more detail in the next section, and training will be offered throughout three sessions in the integrative approach in Part 3.

2.2.2 Promotion of a Healthy Lifestyle Module in the Integrative Approach

Information on the psychoeducational component on healthy and regular habits has been extended with the aim of including the aspects detailed in this section. It is reflected in the corresponding session of integrative psychotherapy included in Part 3.

Mindfulness

Stress is part of life. As discussed previously, some degree of stress can be stimulating to achieve certain goals. However, when the level of stress is maintained, the effects can be detrimental to health. Stress depends not only on the objective situation, but especially on factors related to how we interpret the situation and the resources we believe we have to deal with it. Faced with a stressful situation, the body undergoes a series of physiological reactions that involve the activation of the hypothalamic–pituitary–adrenal axis and the autonomic nervous system. What happens in the stress response is that a real or imagined problem causes the cerebral cortex to send an alarm to the hypothalamus, which then stimulates part of the nervous system to make a series of changes in the body. These include changes in the heart and breathing rates, muscle tension, metabolism and blood pressure, among others. The adrenal glands secrete corticoids which shut down processes such as digestion, growth, tissue repair and the responses of the immune system.

We can be victims of stress and its consequences for physical and mental health or we can learn to better manage those factors that increase our levels of stress with techniques such as cognitive restructuring, diaphragmatic breathing, muscle relaxation and mindfulness, which may contribute to restoring our bodies to their baseline states. Assertiveness, effective problem solving and good time management can also contribute to reducing some tensions. Therefore, there are several strategies we have to manage stress, most of them related to the components that contribute to its appearance and maintenance, as explained at the end of the previous section.

In bipolar disorder, stress can act as a triggering factor for relapses. Faced with this reality, we can adopt an attitude of helplessness and passivity or a more constructive attitude that places us in an active position towards strategies that allow us to handle the stress better. As Kabat-Zinn states in his book *Wherever You Go, There You Are*: 'You can't stop the waves, but you can learn to surf' (Kabat-Zinn 1994, p. 31).

Mindfulness is an approach that has gradually gained strength as a treatment or complement to many interventions aimed at reducing stress and the anxious and depressive symptomatology that often accompanies it. Mindfulness is a mental training technique originating from Eastern contemplative traditions, specifically Buddhism. However, meditation practices and mindfulness skills can be used in a completely secular way. At the heart of mindfulness training is the recognition that it is not the thoughts or emotions experienced that cause suffering; rather, it is the unskilful attempts at dealing with them.

Together with the relevance of improving stress management to reduce the risk of relapses in bipolar disorder, many patients present subsyndromic anxious and depressive symptoms that could be reduced with mindfulness training; the training also seems to improve emotional regulation and attentional performance (Bojic & Becerra 2017; Lovas &

Schuman-Olivier 2018). Furthermore, because mental and emotional states as well as physical sensations can become warning signs before the onset of a relapse, a higher awareness of these signs can facilitate the selection of the most appropriate responses to face them. For all these reasons, mindfulness training has also been incorporated in the integrative approach presented at the end of this book.

2.3.1 Distinctive Aspects of Mindfulness

What Is Mindfulness?

Mindfulness means paying attention in a particular way: on purpose, in the present moment and non-judgementally (Kabat-Zinn 1994). This allows the person to observe and be more aware of thoughts, feelings and physical sensations, which in turn puts the person in a position of responding more skilfully. It therefore means leaving the 'automatic pilot' in which we often operate, understood as the tendency to behave like automatons, without being aware of what is actually happening moment by moment. For example, how many times has it happened to us that we are on vacation and we don't fully enjoy the last few days because we are more aware of returning to work?

As Vicente Simón (2011, p. 135) states, 'Mindfulness is a way of facing what appears in the consciousness with a balanced and equitable attention, without trying to exclude it or cling to it'. Painful experiences generate greater suffering if we resist accepting them. This resistance often manifests itself in the denial of a problem or discomfort derived from the problem, feelings of guilt, rumination about what happened, self-criticism, insistence on thinking about how we would have liked the situation to be or how we should have acted instead of accepting reality as it is. As a consequence, instead of reducing the level of stress, it heightens it. On other occasions, we use behaviours that increase the problem; for example, there are people who resort to using drugs or alcohol, isolate themselves, spend hours distracting themselves with computer games, eat or shop compulsively or stop doing things they previously enjoyed. In short, they try to escape their discomfort using maladaptive coping strategies. Human beings tend to cling to what is pleasant to them and avoid what generates emotions of displeasure. When we resist and do not accept pain, it generates additional discomfort that leads to greater suffering. Thus, we often find that we are fighting with ourselves as we struggle to try to alter the situation and fail to accept the reality that we have a choice about how we can respond. Furthermore, if we observe carefully, the nature of the experience can change. Observing and learning to 'let go' frees us from certain thought patterns and allows us to be less reactive. Unlike the mind, which tends to run forwards into the future or to get stuck in the past, the breath and the body are 'anchors' to the present moment, and therefore represent a very useful resource in the practice of mindfulness, as will be seen.

Sometimes, mindfulness is mistakenly identified as relaxation. However, although in some cases mindfulness exercises can result in relaxation, that is not the aim of the practice. Mindfulness does not pursue (as does relaxation) reaching a certain state or feeling in a certain way, but rather allowing things to be as they are in the present moment, without judging (e.g. 'I'm a disaster', 'I'm no good at this'). Therefore, there is no 'right way' to practise mindfulness; each practice is different and valuable in itself. Mindfulness is an active process during which the person deliberately chooses to pay attention in a certain way. To get to the present moment there is a need to pause and take a look at what is

Table 2.8 Common methods of perception and reaction vs. mindfulness

- 'Automatic pilot' → stop, take a look and consciously choose the response.
- 'Monkey mind' or wandering and distracted mind → focus attention intentionally.
- Mental time travel to the past and the future → focus attention on the present, on the 'here and now'.
- To judge → observe with curiosity, openness and acceptance.
- Focus on the content → focus on the process.
- Endeavour that things 'should' be different → allow things to be as they are.
- Thoughts as realities → thoughts as mental events.
- Avoidance and resistance → 'turn towards', openness and awareness.
- Fight or resignation → acceptance.
- Clinging and controlling → be able to 'let go'.
- 'Doing' mode → 'being' mode.
- Striving and goal-oriented → non-goal attainment or specific state to be achieved, letting go of outcome and expectation.
- Identification with what is observed (getting caught up in the mind with thoughts, emotions) → identification with the observer without 'getting lost' in what is observed (like a scientist).
- Critical attitude, 'should' statements → loving and compassionate attitude towards others and oneself.
- Reactive responses or impulsive problem solving → intentionally choose the most skilful response, problem solving in a less reactive way and from a broader perspective.

happening. Most of the time when we are practising, we have to continually renew our intention to pay attention, over and over again. We have to bring the mind back from its wanderings and pay attention to the breath, the body. It is at the exact moment when you have noticed the mind wandering and you deliberately decide to re-focus that you are being mindful. These features are summarised in Table 2.8.

If we are more conscious, reduce experiential avoidance and increase the ability to distance ourselves and observe with curiosity, we can better regulate the tendency to ruminate, increase the flexibility of attention and decrease the tendency to judge, selecting the responses in a less reactive way. Mindfulness training will therefore allow us to respond to situations with greater freedom of choice and without being carried away by automatic reactions.

Are There Different Types of Interventions?

Although mindfulness can be a component of different approaches, there are two main mindfulness-based interventions: mindfulness-based stress reduction (MBSR) (Kabat-Zinn 1990) and mindfulness-based cognitive therapy (MBCT) (Segal et al. 2001). MBSR was originally designed to help those individuals with chronic physical health conditions exacerbated by stress have a better quality of life by learning to deal more skilfully with those stressful situations that exacerbated their physical symptoms. MBCT was designed to tackle relapse prevention in recurrent depression through the understanding of the processes that maintain depression and that underlie relapse after recovery. It provides the person with alternative methods for teaching decentring skills, training patients to recognise when their mood is deteriorating, and using techniques that would take up limited resources in channels of information processing that normally sustain ruminative thought–affect cycles. MBCT combines elements of mindfulness meditation practice, alongside cognitive techniques to allow individuals to work with and see more clearly patterns of thinking that may be unhelpful or unskilful. However, the emphasis is not directly on the content of the thoughts but rather on changing the relationship established with them (as well as with emotions and physical sensations), which in turn generates a change of perspective. The idea is to observe the thoughts as external events and to be aware of the way we relate to them. It means moving from a focus on content to a focus on process.

The usual approach is through an intervention of 8 weeks' duration, with 2 hours per week accompanied by various types of practice. Throughout the training, the following aspects are worked on:

✓ Recognise the tendency to be on automatic pilot and explore what happens when we are more aware and intentionally focus our attention on what is happening. Some of the practices that allow the person to work on these aspects are meditation of the body, breathing, and the 'raisin exercise' (this illustrates how paying attention intentionally, without judgement, to the way we eat, for example, can transform the experience).

✓ Emphasise the difference between thinking about a sensation versus experiencing it through our senses. For this, the body scan as a practice that emphasises shifting attention to the various parts of the body is a useful way of training in the practice of observing without judging.

✓ Learn that thoughts and emotions are transitory, similar to sounds. A posture of observing how they come and go is promoted, considering them as external events, adopting an attitude of curiosity, kindness and acceptance. It is important to clarify that acceptance should not be understood as resignation. It does not imply renouncing changing things in the future, but rather not resisting the way things are in the here and now. Acceptance allows us to be fully aware of the difficulties and to give ourselves time, if appropriate, to respond skilfully and not automatically. Sometimes doing nothing, allowing the experience to pass, can be the most skilful response. For this, meditation on sounds, thoughts and emotions can be useful.

What Components Come into Play?

Through consciously (intention) bringing awareness (attention) and acceptance (attitude) to the experience in the present moment, we will be better able to use a wider, more adaptive range of coping skills. There is a significant shift in perspective, which is at the heart of the change. As Shapiro et al. (2006) hypothesise, multiple mechanisms may be facilitated by this shift, including (a) self-regulation; (b) values clarification; (c) cognitive, emotional and behavioural flexibility; and (d) exposure.

Hölzel et al. (2011) suggest several components, working synergistically, through which mindfulness meditation exerts its effects. Furthermore, the authors mention neuroimaging data underlying the following components:

1. Attention regulation: sustaining attention on the chosen object; whenever distracted, returning attention to the object. Associated brain areas: anterior cingulate cortex.
2. Body awareness: focus is usually an object of internal experience (sensory experiences of breathing, emotions or other body sensations). Associated brain areas: insula and temporo-parietal junction.

Table 2.9 Assessment instruments

Mindful Attention Awareness Scale (MAAS).
Five Facet Mindfulness Questionnaire (FFMQ).
Toronto Mindfulness Scale (TMS).
Philadelphia Mindfulness Scale (PHLMS).
Experiences Questionnaire (EQ).
MINDSENS composite index, consisting of items from FFMQ and EQ.
Cognitive and Affective Mindfulness Scale–Revised (CAMS–R).
Kentucky Inventory of Mindfulness Skills (KIMS).
Freiburg Mindfulness Inventory (FMI).
Southampton Mindfulness Questionnaire (SMQ).
Mindfulness/Mindlessness Scale (MMS).

3. Emotion regulation:
   - Reappraisal – approaching ongoing emotional reactions in a different way (non-judgementally, with acceptance). Associated brain areas: (dorsal) prefrontal cortex.
   - Exposure, extinction and reconsolidation – exposing oneself to whatever is present in the field of awareness; letting oneself be affected by it; refraining from internal reactivity. Associated brain areas: ventro-medial prefrontal cortex, hippocampus and amygdala.
4. Change in perspective on the self: detachment from identifications with a static sense of self. Associated brain areas: medial prefrontal cortex, posterior cingulate cortex, insula, temporo-parietal junction.

Are There Assessment Instruments?

Table 2.9 presents the main assessment instruments for bipolar disorder. They differ in regard to conceptual aspects and psychometric properties, which have been summarised in the review carried out by Park et al. (2013).

Are There Different Types of Practice?

A crucial aspect of mindfulness training is that both the participants and the instructors should take time every day to practise. The fact that the therapist has regular, first-hand training puts him or her in a better position to understand and respond to the difficulties participants will face. The training sessions involve practising alongside the patients but with a focus on how the participants are doing.

Practice can be formal or informal:

✓ **Formal practice** is that which is done in a regulated way, adopting a specific posture (usually seated) and reserving a specific time of the day to do it (e.g. by using the help of an audio guide, especially at the beginning). Although some manuals recommend devoting 45 minutes a day to formal practice, our experience suggests that some flexibility is desirable, with continuous daily practice being better, even if it is somewhat shorter in length, than practising for a longer time but infrequently.

Some recommendations for formal practice:

1. The setting should be quiet and comfortable, without interruptions and with adequate environmental conditions that facilitate the practice.
2. Wear comfortable clothes and have a light blanket at hand.
3. The regularity of the practice is essential. It is preferable to reserve a fixed time in the agenda for formal practice (e.g. in the morning just before getting up or at night just before going to bed). However, any time is better than nothing. Daily and regular practice produces greater benefits than longer but sporadic practice.
4. The correct attitude during the practice focuses on not having any expectations. It is intended to observe reality as it is, not as we would like it to be. The key is to accept thoughts, emotions and physical sensations, even if they are negative and unpleasant, without judging or criticising oneself for it. Use the mind of the beginner, as if it were the first time we were having the experience, with an attitude of acceptance, openness, curiosity and kindness towards oneself.
5. In breathing meditation, it is not a matter of forcing or changing the breath, but simply observing it as it is at that precise moment.
6. If distracting thoughts, feelings or sensations appear and the mind begins to wander, take note and return it to the anchor point (e.g. breathing).

✓ **Informal practice** can be carried out at any time, applying it to activities of daily life (e.g. brushing teeth, having breakfast, walking). Informal practice allows us to incorporate and generalise what we have been working on in formal practice to our day to day lives.

Practice can be carried out in different ways, but it is basically a matter of consciously directing attention to some internal (e.g. breathing, body sensations, a feeling) or external phenomenon (e.g. sounds, landscape, smells) with an attitude of curiosity, acceptance and openness. Each time the mind moves away from the object to be attended to, we will take note of the thought or stimulus that distracted us, assuming this constant wandering to be the natural way of functioning of our mind. Subsequently, we will kindly direct our attention, again, to the phenomenon attended to. We can also widen or narrow the focus of our attention, as well as alternating the different phenomena we observe.

Table 2.10 is a summary of exercises that can be done in formal and informal practice.

Bringing back the wandering mind requires effort, as in any kind of training (e.g. lifting weights at the gym) but, in a similar way, the more we do it, the easier it becomes. For this reason, we must reinforce the practice and encourage persistence. A good exercise is to set the mobile alarm throughout the day and devote a few minutes to breathing each time it sounds. In some cases, if there are many difficulties, it may be useful to introduce movement, make the practice shorter and increase the time progressively. After completing the practice, feedback is essential. Drawing parallels between what is observed in practice and how we function in our daily lives can reinforce the importance of the exercises.

In order to illustrate some aspects of mindfulness, the use of metaphors is also very helpful. They are an ideal way to respond to the transience of thoughts and other mental events from the perspective of an external observer by means of identifying yourself with the following images: the sky, and observe how mental phenomena arise and vanish like the changing weather or clouds that pass by; a mountain rooted in stillness amidst the constant changes that represent your internal and external experiences; a cinema screen that projects the thoughts that come to your mind; a turbulent lake that calms after a storm, identifying

Table 2.10 Formal and informal practice

Formal practice	Informal practice
– Mindfulness of the breath.	– Washing your face or hands.
– The raisin exercise.	– Having a shower.
– 3-minute breathing space.	– Washing dishes.
– Body scan.	– Going up and downstairs.
– Mindfulness of sounds.	– Brushing your teeth.
– Mindfulness of thoughts.	– Brushing your hair.
– Mindfulness of emotions.	– Getting dressed.
– Sitting meditation.	– Folding your clothes.
– Meditation for giving and receiving love.	– Cooking.
– Walking meditation.	– Mindful eating.
– Yoga alternating with body scan.	– Drinking tea or coffee.
– …	– Driving.
	– Mindful walking.
	– Listening to someone.
	– Playing a musical instrument.
	– Listening to music.
	– …

yourself with the entire body of water so that you become steady and calm below the surface even when it is turbulent on the outside; a train that passes by; actors on a stage. For other practices (e.g. that of walking), it can be interesting to use the metaphor of exploring everything as a child would who is performing the behaviour for the first time or as an alien for whom everything is new, that is, with the beginner's mind. Another resource used to illustrate the nature of mindfulness is poetry (e.g. 'The Guest House,' by Rumi).

Why Is Practice Important?

The experiences offered by practice are a good reflection of the habits of the mind. Being aware of the obstacles that can arise in both types of practice (drowsiness, restlessness, tiredness, boredom, impatience, physical discomfort, distraction caused by anticipation of future events of concern, 'lack of time', self-criticism) provides the opportunity to observe, accept and redirect attention without judging. It is essential to analyse with the participants the difficulties that arise. It is about being aware of the tendency of the mind to wander and become distracted, and to take advantage of the opportunities offered by the practice to deepen and continue practising full consciousness. It is also possible to practise intentionally, carrying these difficulties to the mind in order to increase the ability to handle them when they arise naturally. It should not be forgotten that even resistance to practice gives us information about the habits of our mind. Approaching the practice as an 'experiment' can help in not prejudging and to simply concentrate on exploring the process, fostering an attitude of curiosity. Keeping a diary of frequency, types of practice, duration and observations will allow us to delve deeper and identify whether there are any obstacles that must be considered. As Kabat-Zinn says, the spirit of mindfulness is to practise for its own sake and to take each moment as it comes – pleasant or unpleasant, good or bad – and then work with that because it is what is present now.

Both formal and informal practices allow the person to:

✓ Be aware of the mind's tendency to wander.

✓ Be aware that he or she often operates on 'automatic pilot'.

✓ Train the mind to focus and pay attention.

✓ Be more aware of real experience, which makes it easier to make better decisions.

✓ Realise how the mind works (clinging to what it considers pleasant, fleeing from what is unpleasant, establishing judgements, associations between thoughts and certain emotions, reactions, etc.) and thus allowing the person to change the way he or she relates to these mental events.

✓ Note how paying attention to the experience changes its nature.

✓ Be more aware of negative thoughts and moods, allowing the person to handle them better and generating greater control over the behaviour.

✓ See how thoughts, emotions and physical sensations are transitory, and not take them as 'absolute truths' that require an immediate response. This will allow the person to select more appropriate responses.

✓ Reduce avoidance of experience through sustained exposure.

✓ Reduce rumination or repetitive thinking.

✓ Understand that both the breath (observing how it flows naturally, without attempting to force it) and the focus on the body are crucial, as they are used as a link to the present moment.

- Regarding breathing:

  o It allows us to anchor our attention 'here and now'.

  o It is present 24 hours a day.

  o It does not produce attachment.

  o It contributes to increasing the awareness of our body, where the breath can be observed (nostrils, chest, belly).

  o It is linked to emotional states and can facilitate their regulation, as well as the control of rumination or repetitive thoughts.

  o It represents a bridge between the automatic and the voluntary.

- Regarding the body:

  o It provides another perspective from which to contemplate the experience, a different point of view from which to relate to thoughts and emotions.

  o Emotions have bodily components, and bodily sensations can influence and in turn be affected by thoughts, emotions and behaviours.

  o Sensations are an indicator of mood; therefore, paying attention to the body gives us information about our emotional state and can help to better regulate emotions.

  o It allows us to train the mind using the body and allows attention to be diverted from the 'mind' to the body.

  o Paying attention to sensations of which we have not been aware modifies our experience.

○ Bringing awareness to the body can guide us to introduce beneficial aspects – for example, intentionally changing posture or facial expression helps to change one of the components of the 'mental modality' that keeps us trapped in a certain emotional state.

○ Body awareness facilitates the exposure and management of pain or physical discomfort, allowing us to accept the fear of pain or associated discomfort. If it emerges, it must be observed with curiosity and openness, as well as the chain of associated thoughts and emotions. However, it should be borne in mind that people with negative emotions about their body may perceive this exercise as more aversive. It is important to empathise and validate these sensations, but encourage people to perform the exercise with a curious and kind attitude, open to whatever comes up, or address the issue in a deeper way if necessary.

Why Incorporate Mindfulness into an Integrative Approach to Bipolar Disorder?

As discussed in the section on evidence-based psychological treatments, mindfulness itself has not yet been shown (in the few studies conducted) to be useful in preventing relapses of bipolar disorder. However, some studies indicate that it may contribute to improving the anxious and depressive residual symptomatology the person suffering from the illness often presents, as well as to improving emotional regulation. Furthermore, the fact that stress acts as a triggering factor for relapses reinforces the importance of teaching techniques that make it possible to manage stress better in order to avoid its negative consequences. In the introduction to bipolar disorder, it was also stated that several studies have shown that a significant percentage of patients continue to present deficits in attention, memory and executive functions even when euthymic. Therefore, incorporating mindfulness as a component of a treatment programme is fully justified if we consider a comprehensive approach to the management of this disease. Individuals with bipolar disorder might find mindfulness training particularly helpful, as it is often 'attachment' to the 'good' feelings of hypomania that can lead the individual to relapse. Mindfulness teaches us to welcome all the emotions we experience in the same way and consequently allows the person to be less reactive to emotions and avoid automatic behaviours. Training can help the person become more aware of thoughts, emotions and body sensations related to hypomania/mania or depression and respond less automatically. Early detection of the first warning signs from a more objective perspective will allow the selection of the most appropriate responses to slow down the progression of symptoms. In the case of depression, for example, being aware of the temporary nature of all mental phenomena allows for a higher level of tolerance for unpleasant internal states and choosing the best response to cope with them.

Although there is a need for more research on mindfulness training for bipolar disorder, it can be expected that mindfulness may help individuals with bipolar disorder in different ways, including the following:

✓ Greater acceptance of the disorder and about some uncertainty regarding its course.

✓ Better awareness of changes in mood.

✓ More awareness of changes in the state of mind (speed of thought, etc.).

✓ More awareness of changes in bodily sensations.

✓ More awareness of first warning signs of relapses and activating appropriate strategies.
✓ Better ability to recognise stress and acting accordingly to reduce its harmful effects.
✓ Preventive factor.
✓ Improving communication with family and friends, also concerning issues related to the illness.
✓ Training attention networks for improved focus and concentration.
✓ Better management of anxiety.
✓ Improved management of depressive subsyndromic symptoms.
✓ Reducing the rumination that often accompanies depressive symptomatology.
✓ Improvement of emotional self-regulation.
✓ Substitution of automatic responses (impulsivity, reactivity) by more adaptive strategies.
✓ Feeling more compassionate towards oneself and others.
✓ Being more connected with the present moment.
✓ Increasing the sensation of well-being.

Murray and collaborators (2017) suggest the relevance and clinical implications that regulation of attention and emotions, body awareness and change in one's perspective have on bipolar disorder. They highlight how these aspects can potentially affect the improvement of neurocognition and socio-occupational functioning; the detection and management of prodromes; emotional, cognitive and behavioural regulation; the avoidance of progression to relapses; the management of comorbidities and symptoms such as anxiety; the improvement of quality of life; and the reduction of self-stigma. Some of these themes emerged in a qualitative study in which participants with bipolar disorder highlighted the benefits of the following aspects: focusing on what is present; awareness of mood state/ change; acceptance; mindfulness practice in different mood states; reduction/stabilisation of negative affect; relating differently to negative thoughts; and reduction of the impact of mood state (Chadwick et al. 2011).

2.3.2 Mindfulness Module in the Integrative Approach

All the foregoing aspects of the effects of mindfulness justify the fact that the integrative approach includes three mindfulness training sessions, which are elaborated in Part 3. On the basis of these sessions, not only material (e.g. audios, links, apps, books, weekly practice logs) will be provided to promote sustained repeated practice, but also a brief mindfulness practice will be included in the remainder of the sessions.

Cognitive and Functional Remediation

Cognitive functions encompass the mental processes that take place in the brain, in the central nervous system, related to thinking, decision making, planning, paying attention, remembering. In recent years, the increasing prevalence of dementia in the general population has led to a growing interest in stimulating cognitive functions. This greater awareness of the importance of preserving and improving our cognitive functions has been accompanied by a proliferation of brain training programmes, especially with the expansion of new technologies. Even so, neuropsychological rehabilitation and its application in different pathologies have been in use for more than a century. While different assessments and treatment procedures for brain injury began to be developed in the 1970s, neuropsychological evaluations acquired a relevant status in the world of psychiatry in the late twentieth century, with a particular focus on schizophrenia. Currently, the study of cognitive functioning has been extended to other psychiatric illnesses, especially affective disorders such as bipolar disorder and depression.

Research in the field of bipolar disorder started later, as the illness was traditionally considered to be more cognitively and functionally preserved. However, evidence has shown that both cognitive and functional impairments are also intrinsic characteristics of bipolar disorder, although to a lesser extent than in schizophrenia. Importantly, dysfunction may even be present in euthymic patients. Bipolar disorder is considered a highly disabling illness in some cases, placing a great burden on both patients and the health system, ranking among the top 20 causes of disability in the world (Vos et al. 2012).

Is There Cognitive Impairment in Bipolar Disorder?

Cognitive impairment affects approximately 30–60% of patients with bipolar disorder, to a greater or lesser extent, in both type I and in type II (traditionally considered as 'less severe' although this is not always the case). Deficits are manifested mainly in the cognitive domains of attention, memory (especially verbal memory) and executive functions, with memory and concentration difficulties being the most frequent complaints (Martinez-Aran et al. 2004). Patients usually complain about not being able to enjoy leisure activities as they previously did, such as reading or going to the cinema, not remembering things previously explained to them, forgetting an appointment and so on. The term 'executive functions' is not part of the vocabulary of the general population; therefore, complaints are not as closely related to these functions. However, in a clinical practice a significant proportion of patients recognise difficulties related to those functions that involve planning and organising activities and the ability to adapt to changing or competitive environments (e.g. 'It's very difficult to get organised', 'I start many tasks at home and leave them all

Table 2.11 Relationship between cognitive functions and daily activities

Cognitive function	Definition	Examples of daily activities
Attention and processing speed	Ability that allows us to be oriented towards a certain stimulus or situation and ignore the rest. Time it takes to produce an answer.	– Driving, reading a book, watching a movie. – Reacting quickly if we see an object falling. – Quickly check to see whether we correctly completed a document with our personal data.
Memory	Processes involved in coding, storing and retrieving information (remembering past experiences, general knowledge acquired, recognising previously learned information, implicit or procedural learning, remembering things to do in the future).	Declarative memory: – Remembering a shopping list or names of famous people. – Remembering where a dress was bought or details of a trip. Working memory: – Remembering a phone number just after it was heard. – Calculating the change for purchases. – Memorising dishes to serve and knowing which diners each one corresponds to.
Executive function	Functions needed to plan, guide, review, regulate and evaluate our behaviours in order to adapt effectively to our environment.	– Planning and organising a birthday party. – Solving an unforeseen problem. – Decision making.
Social cognition	Abilities that allow us to process information from social situations, understand and interpret the emotions and intentions of others.	– Recognising whether a friend is sad through facial expressions. – Putting ourselves in someone else's position and understanding why they act in a certain way.

half-done', 'I'm late for appointments'). It is worth mentioning that cognitive impairment is highly heterogeneous among patients with bipolar disorder, so that not all individuals present with cognitive difficulties. Memory deficits may be more prevalent in some patients, while in others executive functioning issues predominate. Follow-up studies are still scarce and not clear enough about the progression of cognitive impairment in bipolar disorder; some studies indicate that cognition tends to remain rather stable over time (Mora et al. 2016; Torrent et al. 2012). Table 2.11 outlines the main cognitive functions that are affected in bipolar disorder along with some examples of everyday activities.

In recent years, social cognition has acquired greater relevance. Social cognition is a set of processes that allows us to process information in social situations and therefore understand and predict the behaviour of others, as well as draw inferences from what we perceive in others and make decisions based on this information. Social cognition encompasses different dimensions such as the recognition of emotions, empathy and theory of mind. The latter refers to the ability to infer both one's own feelings and those of others from data perceived during social interactions. Although available evidence is scarce, it suggests that patients suffering from bipolar disorder may present deficits in theory of mind, even when they are remitted (Bora et al. 2016).

Why Are Cognitive Difficulties Observed in Bipolar Disorder?

Thought processes take place in the brain, and the disease also originates in and affects the functioning of some areas of the brain related to these cognitive processes. The limbic system is one of these. Some structures of this system are related to emotions, while other areas are more involved in cognitive processing. For example, the hippocampus and the amygdala play an important role in memory. The latter seems to be specifically involved in the storage of information based on its emotional content and is also implicated in the learning of emotional behaviours.

Several clinical and pharmacological factors may be directly or indirectly related to cognitive functioning in bipolar disorder (Figure 2.7). According to numerous studies, the variables most affecting cognitive functioning include the following:

- Chronicity (number of years of illness).
- Number of affective episodes, primarily those manic episodes which produce greater neurotoxic effects on the brain.
- The subclinical symptomatology (residual symptoms that do not meet sufficient criteria to be considered an affective episode), more specifically the depressive type.

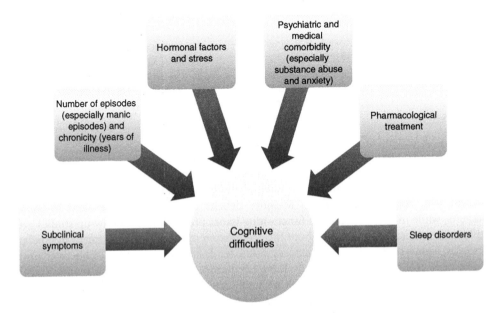

Figure 2.7 Factors affecting cognition.

- Hormonal factors. A rise in cortisol (a hormone released in response to stress) level is usually common in both depressive and manic episodes. Hypercortisolaemia maintained for prolonged periods could damage structures related to memory, such as the hippocampus.
- Sleep disturbances. Good sleep routines are crucial to avoid future relapses. In addition, sleep deprivation increases difficulties with memory and concentration. Sleep is involved in the processing of experiences and facilitates the consolidation of memory, strengthening the neuronal connections that form our memories.
- Pharmacological treatments. It is difficult to control the influence of medication given the complexity of bipolar disorder treatment, characterised by the wide availability of medications as well as by a fairly frequent use of polytherapy. It has been shown that some drugs may affect cognition (e.g. topiramate), while others may even be neuroprotective (e.g. lithium and valproate). Studies with small samples have observed cognitive deficits in drug-free patients as well as at very early stages of the disease. Therefore, cognitive impairment in bipolar disorder would not be explained simply as a side effect of medication but also as a consequence of the disease.
- Comorbidity with other medical conditions is quite common in patients suffering from bipolar disorder. Among psychiatric comorbidities, anxiety disorders and substance abuse in particular stand out, and both conditions may significantly contribute to the magnitude of cognitive dysfunction. Therefore, identifying and treating these comorbidities will be crucial to improving cognitive performance.

Finally, the concept of cognitive reserve, initially developed in the field of neurology, reflects the capacity of an adult brain to resist brain pathology in order to minimise clinical manifestations and compensate cognitive impairment (Stern 2009). This concept is used to explain why some individuals function better than others in the presence of brain pathology. Cognitive reserve is fundamentally related to three factors: the pre-morbid intelligence quotient (IQ), the level of academic and educational achievements, and leisure activities. Variables such as lifestyle, diet, intellectual activity or ability to speak several languages also have a significant influence on cognitive reserve. While the IQ would represent the most innate and stable characteristic of this concept, the academic and educational achievements, as well as leisure activities and lifestyle, would be potentially modifiable components. Therefore, cognitive reserve may be enriched or boosted by exercising our brain with the accumulation of knowledge through continuous educational training and intellectual and cultural activities, such as learning new skills or engaging in leisure activities that are mentally challenging (reading, photography, sewing, gardening, writing, playing a musical instrument, learning a new language, etc.). Enhancing cognitive reserve may allow people to cope better with a neurological or psychiatric illness or age-related brain changes. Therefore, the objective will be to find new ways to stimulate the brain with enjoyable activities and learning at the same time, over the life course and not only at early ages. In the past 5 years, several articles have been published pointing out an association between cognitive reserve, psychosocial functioning and performance in specific cognitive domains (Anaya et al. 2016; Forcada et al. 2014).

Why Is an Intervention Aimed at Improving Cognitive Function Important?

Cognitive impairment in mental illness is a key factor in therapeutic management and prognosis. In this sense, multiple findings have demonstrated the value of cognitive variables on global psychosocial functioning, that is, the role that cognition exerts on work or academic performance or even on social relationships. For example, attentional and concentration problems may generate difficulties in maintaining a conversation with friends which, in the long term, can lead to social isolation. Difficulties in organisation and time management can lead to difficulties in maintaining the pace of work, which, over time, may imply choosing an easier job or making it impossible to have regular work. In fact, many patients with bipolar disorder report lasting difficulties after hospitalisation. Although today there is no doubt about the role of cognition in general functioning, other factors such as variables related to the clinical course of the disease (e.g. age at onset, number of episodes) and sociodemographic factors (e.g. gender, age, diagnostic subtype) also influence psychosocial functioning.

Besides the disability that cognitive deficits produce by themselves, another important reason to treat cognitive deficits is the limitation they place on patients' ability to benefit from other types of psychosocial interventions.

Finally, as has been mentioned, enhancing cognitive reserve can slow down the ageing process.

Therefore, cognition will be a main target in the treatment of the disease, especially to minimise the impact of cognitive deficits on daily functioning.

How Can We Prevent or Improve Cognitive Impairment in Bipolar Disorder?

As shown in Figure 2.8, there are different approaches to consider in order to prevent or improve cognitive dysfunction in bipolar disorder. First, as mentioned, psychotherapeutic programmes such as psychoeducation allow patients and family members to acquire better knowledge, awareness and acceptance of the illness, thereby enhancing treatment adherence and other fundamental tips for preventing new affective episodes. Psychoeducation is always complementary to effective pharmacotherapy in order to prevent future relapses and achieve affective stability. It will also be important to treat those comorbidities that may affect the course of the disorder and cognitive processes. The pharmacological regimen for each patient should include those therapeutic options that affect cognition as little as possible. Today there is an increasing interest in developing drugs to enhance cognitive function, known as pro-cognitive drugs, in the fields of both neurological and psychiatric diseases. Even so, none has been approved yet as a pro-cognitive enhancer for severe mental disorders such as schizophrenia or bipolar disorder. However, ongoing studies are likely to offer hopeful results for some of these pro-cognitive agents in the near future.

Conversely, another therapeutic option would be establishing cognitive remediation programmes to treat these deficits. However, whereas many studies have been published and different cognitive interventions have been developed in schizophrenia, research has, until the past decade, been scarce in the area of bipolar disorder and is still in its early stages. The section on scientific evidence contains a brief description of the main studies on cognitive remediation with samples composed exclusively of patients with bipolar disorder.

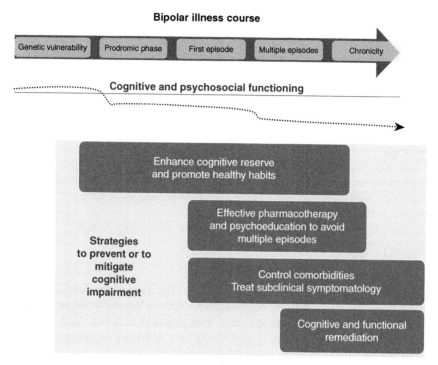

Figure 2.8 Strategies to prevent or mitigate cognitive dysfunction.

Although cognitive remediation has been proposed as an effective treatment tool in the field of psychiatric illnesses, it was not until 2010 that a clear definition concerning this type of intervention was given by the Cognitive Remediation Experts Workshop. This group of experts defined cognitive remediation as an intervention based on behavioural training, aimed at improving cognitive processes (attention, memory, executive functions, social cognition or metacognition) with the aim of achieving a durable and generalised improvement (Wykes & Spaulding 2011). Other authors, however, define cognitive remediation as a treatment to improve neurocognitive functioning, involving a learning process and attempts to influence psychosocial functioning (Penadés & Gastó 2010). Therefore, cognitive remediation is not just a specific intervention isolated from cognitive processes.

The functional remediation programme, a therapeutic intervention designed by the Barcelona Bipolar and Depressive Disorders Unit to treat the cognitive and functional impairment associated with bipolar disorder, is explained in more detail in the following section.

2.4.1 Distinctive Aspects of Functional Remediation for Patients with Bipolar Disorders

What Is Functional Remediation?

The development of functional remediation represents a scientific effort to build a psychotherapeutic intervention aimed at solving the functional problems of patients with bipolar disorder facing the cognitive deficits associated with the illness, adapted to the

Table 2.12 Distinctive aspects of functional remediation

Functional remediation implies . . .
– Educational and metacognitive components about cognitive deficits associated with the disorder and its impact on daily functioning.
– A neurocognitive–behavioural approach that includes modelling techniques, role-playing, self-instructions, positive reinforcement and metacognition.
– That it is aimed not only at cognitive improvement but also at psychosocial functioning.
– Training in strategies to improve performance in attention, memory and executive functions domains.
– Training of impaired functions and implementation of compensatory strategies.
– Learning ecological neurocognitive strategies and techniques to be transferred to daily life.
– Training in communication skills and stress reduction techniques for managing stressful situations and enhancing autonomy.
– Involving the family in facilitating the implementation and practice of the techniques learned by participants.

characteristics and specific needs of this population. The basis of functional remediation is to achieve a real transfer of the new neurocognitive skills or learned strategies to daily life in the context of a highly ecological approach with practical exercises. This programme is based on the neurocognitive–behavioural model that addresses neurocognition and psychosocial aspects (Table 2.12).

How and When Is Functional Remediation Implemented?

Functional remediation was designed to take place in a group format (about 10 patients per group), although it can also be implemented individually, with minor modifications. The group format can help foster social relationships, and has the benefit of reaching a larger number of people. It also promotes a sense of equality, wherein participants can share similar experiences and learn from each other about the use of different techniques and strategies. However, the intervention may also offer some advantages when it is delivered individually, as the possibility of establishing personalised objectives takes into account needs, capacities and the patient's environment, including tasks and activities linked to these goals. The connection between the programme and objectives linked to the patient's real life, such as the working environment, social life or autonomy in daily tasks, will help the patient to perceive participation in these programmes as relevant and useful.

It is highly recommended that the intervention is conducted when patients are euthymic, or with subclinical symptomatology that does not meet the criteria for an affective episode, so that their capacity for learning is optimal.

What Are the Components of a Functional Remediation Programme for Patients with Bipolar Disorders?

Functional remediation was tested in the context of a randomised, blind clinical trial, which is the highest standard by which to test any pharmacological or psychotherapeutic treatment. The results of this study (Torrent et al. 2013) were published in the *American Journal of Psychiatry*, a high-impact journal, showing that functional remediation made patients

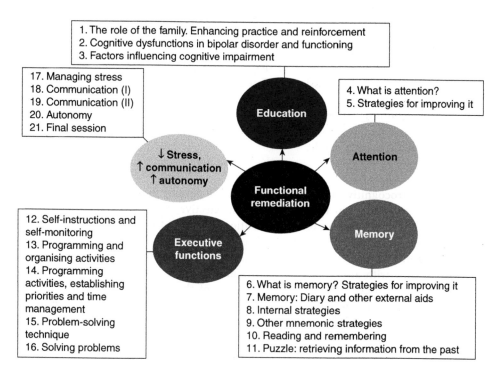

Figure 2.9 Sessions of the group functional remediation programme for bipolar disorders (Barcelona Bipolar and Depressive Disorders Unit).

function better, especially in the interpersonal and occupational domains. *Functional Remediation for Bipolar Disorder* is recommended as a guide for implementing functional remediation (Vieta et al. 2014, www.cambridge.org).

The functional remediation intervention consists of 21 weekly sessions, 90 minutes each, grouped into five blocks (Figure 2.9). Each session is supported by a set of PowerPoint slides to display the contents and materials for participants. Homework is assigned at the end of each session to reinforce and promote strategies in patients' daily lives.

The following provides a brief description of the five functional remediation modules, together with some guidelines for each:

1. Education

The first module contains three sessions devoted to providing basic information on neuro-cognitive processes. The main objective of these sessions is to explain the nature of the relationship between disease progression and neurocognitive dysfunction. Not all patients are aware of their cognitive difficulties and repercussions in their daily functioning. Two sessions deal with educating or training participants in neurocognitive impairment associated with the illness and those factors influencing their cognitive performance. In addition, there is a brief explanation concerning some positive factors (e.g. diet, physical exercise, sleep regularity) and negative factors (e.g. number of relapses, substance abuse, poor treatment adherence) that may interfere with neurocognitive performance and functioning, and over which patients may exert a certain amount of control. Dysfunctional beliefs and prejudices related to patients' neurocognitive deficits may make them feel anxious or embarrassed. In this regard, some myths (e.g. 'The medication causes the cognitive deficits', 'There is greater intellectual capacity during an episode of mania') are discussed to help with the process of destigmatisation. Although the intervention is addressed to patients, the first session is offered to family members in order to explain the objectives of the intervention and clarify any questions related to neurocognitive deficits and their implications in patients' daily lives. In this family session, it is recommended that relatives encourage the patient to attend the sessions and to do the homework, boosting their autonomy whenever possible.

2. Attention

Training in neurocognitive functions begins in the second module with two sessions devoted to training different types of attention: selective, sustained and divided attention. After a brief introduction to what attention means and which aspects of daily life are compromised by deficits in this area (e.g. losing the thread of a conversation, not remembering the name of an interlocutor, difficulties in following a film plot), several strategies to cope with attentional difficulties are provided and practised by means of different exercises to consolidate their use. Some of the guidelines explained involve taking breaks during attention-straining tasks, limiting tasks rather than attempting to multitask several activities, avoiding starting new activities before others are completed, eliminating distractions in the environment, and so on. Within this block, participants are also trained to regulate attentional capacity through the use of self-instruction, a resource based on internal language to guide self-behaviour (e.g. when faced with a task, patients will look for external clues to detect whether attention has been lost by using phrases such as 'Am I paying attention to what I'm doing?', 'I've lost my train of thought ... I'm going to refocus on what I was doing'). Patients are also encouraged to train their attentional capacity by means of a word search, looking for differences between two images, mental calculation tasks, Sudoku, and so on. The objective is to propose a wide range of strategies, so that each patient can adopt those which personally work best for him or her.

3. Memory

One of the main complaints made by patients with bipolar disorder as well as one of the most replicated deficits in the scientific literature is memory; hence, this module includes a greater number of sessions. Participants are trained in internal strategies to enhance the process of encoding to help retrieval memory, that is, to learn to adequately organise new information so that access to information will be more effective. This group of techniques (such as association, categorisation and visual imagery) promotes more profound processing to make new information more meaningful. These mnemonic techniques are practised with different exercises, with the objective being to later transfer them to patients' daily routines. Because memory difficulties often involve problems with remembering the names of people, some techniques to improve this are provided. Patients are also trained in the use of external aids that refer to instruments or tools to reduce the impact of cognitive deficits on daily life and compensate impaired functions (e.g. diary, clock alarms, information and communication technologies (ICTs), calendar). The objective is not only to enhance or optimise the use of external aids but also to destigmatise their use. Special emphasis is placed on the use of a diary (notebook, smartphone), because it will improve patients' independence and involve mental effort, which may help to enhance the encoding and retrieval of information. Some strategies that allow the reconstruction of information from the past, such as better organising memories with well-classified, ordered and labelled photos, recordings, and videos of important events, are also provided. Finally, one session within this block is dedicated to reacquiring the reading habit, lost by a significant proportion of patients given their difficulties in their ability to maintain concentration or to remember what was previously read. Patients are encouraged to read a specified number of chapters of a book every week, and to respond to a series of questions to evaluate their level of understanding. Patients also must choose a piece of news in the newspaper and track it every week.

4. Executive Functions

This module includes five sessions focused on executive functions, those functions that allow us to constantly adapt to changes required by the environment. Activities within this module promote the use of several strategies to enhance planning to meet goals, programme day-to-day activities, focus on time management, and adapt to unforeseen events, alongside training in problem-solving techniques. This takes place in an ecological setting to achieve a real transfer of these strategies to daily life functioning. Problem-solving training will translate into greater efficacy in coping with problems, as well as reducing stress and negative thoughts ('I can't do anything', 'This has no solution', 'I'm not able to manage this situation'). After the different steps of the problem-solving technique have been explained, the method is practised using an example. Then, participants are encouraged to train using their own problems in situ with the aim of familiarising themselves with the method and learning to use a procedure that works for them to increase their skills to solve problems that may arise in their daily lives.

5. Stress, Communication and Autonomy

Module 5, the final module, includes sessions that integrate different aspects related to stress management, such as improving communication and interpersonal relationships, and some well-known techniques to reduce stress, such as diaphragmatic breathing and progressive muscle relaxation. As has been mentioned previously, exposure to continued stress may lead to negative consequences (physical and psychological) and plays an important role as a possible trigger of relapses. Therefore, it will be useful to provide patients with different tools to better manage stress and anxiety. Concerning communication, sessions are focused on providing guidelines to establish appropriate communication, promoting assertiveness and reflective listening. Improving communication skills also contributes to effective problem solving and better management of anxiety and discomfort. The penultimate session, which is focused on improving autonomy and functioning, is conducted by a social worker to provide patients with information concerning activities that may be done in the community, volunteer services, civic centres and the like as well as relevant issues and resources related to individual occupational situations (pensions, disability, etc.). In general, all these sessions aim to empower the patients' autonomy, encouraging them to do as many tasks as possible by themselves: control of medication, mobile phone applications, administrative tasks, and so on. To close, the last session consists of a summary of all the programme sessions and a brief evaluation of the intervention by patients.

2.4.2 Cognitive and Functional Enhancement Module in the Integrative Approach

The cumulative experience over the past 10 years of implementing the functional remediation programme has served as a guide to select the content considered essential to be included in the brief integrative psychotherapy for bipolar disorder, as is shown Part 3. The integrative approach includes a cognitive and functional enhancement module which encompasses the main strategies and techniques used to improve attentional capacity, memory and executive functions, such as planning and organising activities and time management. Some strategies such as problem-solving techniques and training in communication skills, that are also used in other programmes previously mentioned, will be incorporated within this module.

Introduction to the Integrative Approach

Why Is an Integrative Approach Necessary?

As has been pointed out in the introduction, not only does bipolar disorder have a clinical impact but it can also affect other important areas in the lives of people who suffer from it, and their significant others. Therefore, the treatment of the disease should be comprehensive, taking into consideration different areas influenced by the illness. The sessions presented here, written in an informative way to be shared with those suffering from the illness, aim to cover clinical aspects and issues related to physical health, cognitive and psychosocial functioning, and the enhancement of well-being and quality of life. In order to address all these areas, the integrative approach was designed based on a combination of different psychological treatments previously described. Some contents of psychoeducation for patients have been combined with a session for family members, and complemented with aspects related to health promotion, mindfulness training and strategies for cognitive and functional enhancement, always adjunctive to pharmacological treatment. Therefore, the programmes represent the pillars on which the different modules of the integrative treatment were built. In order to make it more generalisable to clinical practice, in the integrative approach these components have been combined in a shorter format, facilitating implementation in mental health centres and hospitals as well in the field of research.

To Whom Is the Integrative Approach Directed?

The integrative approach is aimed at people with bipolar disorder in pharmacological treatment who are stable or have subsyndromic or subclinical symptoms, without therefore meeting the criteria of an acute episode. For this programme, people with other associated psychiatric illnesses (e.g. anxiety disorder) will not be excluded, with the exception of active drug abuse/dependence.

How Are the Sessions Organised?

The intervention can be carried out in either individual or group format.

In the event that the sessions are held in groups, the programme has been structured as a total of twelve 90-minute sessions convening once a week. It is convenient for attendees to form a semicircle around the therapist and co-therapist to facilitate more fluid and direct communication, favouring visual contact and interaction. To illustrate the contents of the sessions, a black- or whiteboard will be necessary as well as a projector or screen as audiovisual support for the presentation of slides in the cognitive enhancement module.

It is recommended that the groups be balanced, being homogeneous enough to create a feeling of identification but with a certain heterogeneity that is enriching. Generally, the sessions are structured by dedicating the first few minutes to holding an informal conversation in which possible incidents and doubts that may have arisen from the last encounter are discussed, and practical exercises (if any) are reviewed or the practice is introduced (e.g. in the sessions about mindfulness and those that follow). Subsequently, the topic of the day is addressed, covering the main objectives of each session with flexibility while encouraging participation and discussion. The formulation of questions that guide the contents, rounds and the use of exercises will encourage the participation of every member of the group, always in a context of acceptance of the degree of involvement and the amount of time that everyone needs. After each session, a summary of the topic worked on is delivered; this material is presented in this section.

If an individual format is used, then the objectives and contents can be personalised and perhaps worked on in more than one session if necessary.

What Is the Role of the Therapist?

It is essential that the therapist has updated knowledge about bipolar disorder, as well as clinical experience in the management of this disease and training in the techniques used and specific components of the integrative approach such as mindfulness. The therapist should have interpersonal skills that foster an atmosphere of empathy, dialogue and trust.

The therapist should be familiar with and comfortable with a group format. From the outset, some general and communication rules should be discussed and emphasised, such as the importance of participants listening to each other and taking turns so that members can express themselves. The therapist should make the sessions lively to maintain attention and encourage the participation of all the attendees. The use of humour on certain occasions can be used to discharge a potentially tense atmosphere, even when serious issues are addressed. Establishing a participatory interaction in which the therapist is directive when appropriate, knowing how to set limits if needed and bringing the discussion back on track with flexibility will allow the objectives set out in each session to be met and allow sufficient time for discussion.

The therapist should be skilful enough to take advantage of the opportunity offered by the group context to correct erroneous beliefs and dismantle myths derived from stigmatisation. In addition, the modelling provided by group work allows the therapist to reinforce and teach the most effective coping strategies. The group can promote awareness of the illness, enrich the contents through the exchange of experiences, incorporate exercises such as role-playing in certain sessions such as communication skills training. A group context is also stimulating in terms of the feedback derived from the practice of exercises such those performed in mindfulness training.

It is recommended there be a co-therapist who plays an active role, whose interventions complement the contents offered by the lead therapist, in addition to facilitating the effective handling of difficult situations that may arise in certain group dynamics. Group work is very stimulating, but it is not exempt from delicate or tense situations, whose potentially toxic atmosphere can be reduced if the objectives and rules of the group are made clear from the beginning and are shared by the participants. If an adequate evaluation has been made, if realistic expectations have been established, if the rules of the group have been clearly stated and if a positive atmosphere of acceptance and respect is generated, then the group will coalesce in a climate of safety.

It is important that, whether the sessions are carried out in an individual or group format, the therapist encourages the participants to perform exercises at home that allow them to deepen the practice, intensifying its effects. For this reason, after each thematic block it is advisable to provide websites, mobile phone applications, readings and other resources that complement what has been worked on in the sessions. Given the rapid progress in this area, the therapist should update this information regularly.

What Sessions Does the Programme Include?

Table 3.1 summarises the programme's 12 once-a-week, 90-minute sessions. As mentioned, the integrative approach consists of psychoeducation for the patient, including a session aimed exclusively at family members. In addition, the promotion of regular and healthy habits, training in mindfulness, and resources and strategies for cognitive and functional enhancement are worked on.

Table 3.1 Integrative approach sessions

1.	Bipolar Disorder: Causes and Triggers.
2.	Symptoms of Bipolar Disorder: Early Detection of Warning Signs and Early Action.
3.	Treatment of Bipolar Disorder and Therapeutic Adherence.
4.	Regularity of Habits and a Healthy Lifestyle.
5.	Psychoeducation Directed at Family Members: Family and Bipolar Disorder.
6.	Mindfulness I: Automatic Pilot versus Awareness.
7.	Mindfulness II: Habits of the Mind and the Importance of the Body.
8.	Mindfulness III: Thoughts and Emotions.
9.	Cognitive and Functional Enhancement: Attention and Memory.
10.	Cognitive and Functional Enhancement: Executive Functions.
11.	Problem-Solving Skills Training.
12.	Assertiveness and Communication Skills.

Contents of the Integrative Approach

The following sections present the material worked on in each of the sessions, adapted for delivery to the participants. As mentioned, each thematic block will be complemented with additional information (constantly updated) in the form of mobile applications, links, audios and literature so that members can go deeper into the practice of the components on which they have worked.

3.2.1 Bipolar Disorder: Causes and Triggers

Normally, mood tends to be stable and may vary slightly depending on external factors. In **bipolar disorder**, however, there is an **alteration of the mechanisms that regulate mood states**. In a somewhat simplistic way, it can be said that most of these structures are located in the limbic system, the area of the brain in charge of acting, much as a thermostat works in a house (we could speak of a kind of 'moodstat'): maintaining a regular temperature (mood) and activating the structures necessary to maintain the balance. When a person suffers from bipolar disorder, the mood – if there is no adequate treatment – becomes unstable, variable and independent of the environment. Therefore, **people with bipolar disorder have oscillations characterised by periods of elevated mood (hypomania or mania) and periods of depression, alternating with periods of stability (euthymia)**, as Figure 3.1 shows. Both the intensity and the frequency of such fluctuations vary from person to person. The intensity of the mood elevation determines the type of bipolar disorder: type I bipolar disorder (at least one manic episode) or type II (hypomania and depression). Proper adherence to pharmacological treatment and a series of behavioural patterns can help to make the oscillations less frequent and less intense, and even prevent them.

Therefore, bipolar disorder is a **chronic** (lifelong) and **recurrent** (episodes tend to happen again) illness, but this does not mean that it cannot be controlled. It is a chronic but treatable disease. That is, it is not 'curable', but proper treatment combined with a healthy lifestyle can help keep it stable.

Bipolar disorder has existed throughout history and has similar prevalence rates in all countries, demonstrating that it is a 'universal' disease, not at all linked to cultural or social determinants. Bipolar disorder, in its various forms, affects approximately **4% of the general population**. In the event that a parent suffers from the disease, the risk of his or her son or daughter having a bipolar disorder would be about 10%. The disease can manifest at any time, although its onset is most often **around the age of 20**, and its start in adolescence is also common.

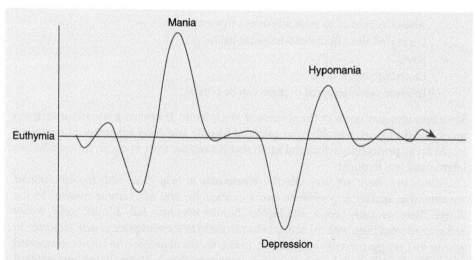

Figure 3.1 Types of mood episodes in bipolar disorder.

Bipolar disorder **does not change the personality** of the individual who suffers from it. Although during episodes of depression or euphoria the symptoms may suggest that the personality has indeed changed, when the episode remits, it will be possible to verify that the personality remains unchanged. Therefore, bipolar disorder is not an alteration of character or personality. We should not say, 'I am bipolar' but instead 'I have a bipolar disorder'. Bipolar disorder is a disease, not a way of being.

The disease has a **biological basis** and is genetically transmitted. Although the **cause of bipolar disorder is genetic**, there are a number of **environmental factors** that can precipitate relapses and thus **influence the course of the disease**. The occurrence of episodes is determined by the interaction between **genetic vulnerability, biological factors and environmental factors**:

➤ The fact that the cause of this disease is **genetic** means that in individuals with bipolar disorder there is probably a family history of similar forms of the illness, but it is also possible for individuals with no family history of bipolar disorder to manifest the disease.

➤ Regarding **biological** factors involved in the disease, neurotransmitters (e.g. dopamine, serotonin, noradrenaline, acetylcholine) are the substances responsible for transporting information in the brain. Abnormalities in neurotransmitter systems have been associated with mood episodes; medication makes it possible to regulate such dysfunction. Hormonal functioning, among others, also seems to play an important role in the disorder. The mood oscillations that can be caused by the alteration of thyroid hormones should be noted, as should the increased risk of relapse in the postpartum period if the person is without medication because of the significant hormonal changes that occur.

➤ **Environmental** factors are not the cause of bipolar disorder, but can positively or negatively influence the course of the illness. Among the most common relapse triggers are the following:

- Abandonment of or poor adherence to medication.
- Decreased sleep hours and irregular habits.
- Stress.
- Consumption of drugs.
- In some cases, seasonal changes can be critical.

Some episodes may occur in the absence of precipitants. However, a low-stress environment, social support, a healthy and balanced lifestyle and good adherence to treatment would act as **protective** factors and mean that if a relapse were to occur, it would be less intense and less frequent.

Fortunately, there are **very effective treatments** to help those with bipolar disorder remain stable, making it possible to lead a 'normal' life and not become enslaved by the illness. There are many people with bipolar disorder who have fully adapted social, family and interpersonal lives, with the ability to be successful in the workplace as well. However, to achieve this, relapse prevention is essential. In fact, the list of people who have been reported to have bipolar disorder who now occupy an important place in history is very long: political leaders including Churchill and Roosevelt; painters including van Gogh, Gauguin and Pollock; brilliant composers including Schumann and Tchaikovsky; pop and rock stars including Kurt Cobain, Peter Gabriel, Tom Waits, Sting and Mariah Carey; actors including Catherine Zeta-Jones and Stephen Fry; writers including Virginia Woolf, Ernest Hemingway, Charles Baudelaire, Hermann Hesse and Edgar Allan Poe.

There are still many myths about mental illness in our society, so an understanding of the reality of the illness is a first step to correcting erroneous and unfounded beliefs.

Having bipolar disorder does not have to be any more serious than suffering from other chronic illnesses such as asthma or diabetes, as **its potential impact can be mitigated by adequate medication and behavioural patterns that involve regular habits and a healthy lifestyle.**

3.2.2 Symptoms of Bipolar Disorder: Early Detection of Warning Signs and Early Action

The basic difference between normal fluctuations and those typical of the disease is that the former – whether or not caused by external events – tend to disappear after a few hours, while those associated with the disorder, if not treated, tend to worsen with the passage of time. Here we will review the main symptoms of mania, hypomania and depression. **If we are able to recognise their appearance as soon as possible, we can act quickly and avoid the negative consequences associated with them.**

Mania

Manic episodes are characterised by **a distinct period of abnormally and persistently elevated, expansive or irritable mood, and by an increase in activity and energy** over a period of time that can range from a week to several months.

Symptoms of mania:

- Increased activity.
- Elevated mood.

- Decreased need for sleep.
- Loquacity or verbosity (more talkative than usual).
- Acceleration of thoughts.
- Inflated self-esteem.
- Distractibility.
- Increased sex drive.
- Irritability.
- Restlessness or psychomotor agitation.
- Grandiosity or overestimation of one's own capabilities and possibilities (can generate excessive economic costs).
- Excessive involvement in pleasurable activities that have a high potential for painful consequences.
- In some cases, psychotic symptoms can occur, in the form of delusions (firmly held irrational beliefs, e.g. to be in direct contact with a divinity, to have special powers, to be a victim of a conspiracy) and/or hallucinations (alteration in perception, e.g. hearing voices, seeing things that do not exist).

In these episodes, mood disturbance is sufficiently severe to cause marked impairment in normal functioning and may require hospitalisation.

Hypomania

Hypomanic episodes are characterised by a minimum period of 4 days wherein the mood is persistently elevated, expansive or irritable, and is accompanied by an increase in levels of activity or energy. It is clearly recognisable as different from a person's regular mood and functioning. The symptoms of hypomania are similar to those of mania but are less intense. In contrast to mania, in hypomania the change in functioning is not severe enough to cause marked impairment in social or occupational functioning, or to require hospitalisation, and there are no psychotic symptoms.

Depression

Depressive episodes are characterised by a period of at least 2 weeks in which the person shows a **depressed mood or a loss of interest or pleasure in nearly all activities**.
   Some of the following symptoms must also be present:

- Depressed mood. Feelings of sadness, emptiness, hopelessness, depression, or crying for no apparent reason.
- Fatigue or loss of energy.
- Diminished ability to think or concentrate.
- Indecisiveness.
- Loss of interest.
- Changes in sleep patterns (insomnia or hypersomnia).
- Significant changes in appetite/weight.
- Irritability.
- Feelings of worthlessness or excessive or inappropriate guilt.
- Recurrent thoughts of death.

– Suicidal ideation or suicide attempt.
– Decreased sexual desire.
– Psychomotor agitation or retardation.
– In some cases, psychotic symptoms (delusions or hallucinations).

During a depressive episode, the emotions (e.g. indifference, sadness, irritability) as well as thoughts (e.g. negativity, decreased processing speed, changes in attention span, concentration and memory) and behaviour (e.g. agitation/inhibition of movement, social isolation) are affected.

The symptoms cause clinically significant distress or impairment in social, occupational or other important areas of functioning.

Mixed Features

In some cases, both hypomania/mania and depressive episodes may have mixed features, described as the **simultaneous** presence of symptoms of an episode of both depression and mania.

Identification of Prodromes

The first signals of an episode are called **prodromes**. Just as the discomfort and suffering typical of depression usually signal a need for help, during a manic episode the person may not recognise that he or she is ill. In both cases, it is very important to identify the onset of new episodes as early as possible, allowing us to act quickly and therefore avoid relapses and the consequences of mood episodes (e.g. hospitalisations, social and occupational difficulties). **The sooner we detect the first warning signs, the more likely it is that we can avoid the progression of symptoms,** preventing the episode or, if it does occur, making it less intense and less disruptive and so requiring less medication to treat it. In addition, it is not uncommon for a depressive episode to occur after mania, so the prevention of hypomania/mania will also reduce this possible risk, and vice versa.

Drawing up a list of prodromes, if possible with the help of a family member, is extremely useful. The following factors should be taken into account:

– Focus on **behaviours** that can be objectively measured.
  What I do instead of what I think about or how I feel.
– Be present **regularly before** previous episodes.
– Evaluate on a **day-to-day basis.**
– **Look for subtle** changes, because the aim is to detect the warning signs that precede the symptom. For example, in a person who usually sleeps 8 hours, sleeping 4 hours would be a symptom but more discreet changes such as 'waking up before the alarm clock rings' or 'sleeping 7 hours' could be a warning sign.
– **Look for distinctive changes in temperament and usual functioning.** For example, initiating conversations with strangers will not have the same meaning in an extroverted person as in a shy person. In terms of functioning, taking into account what is the usual level of activity will serve as a reference point to assess variations – for example, a person who normally goes to the gym once a week who suddenly starts going more than three times a week. Both qualitative changes (e.g. developing a sudden, intense new passion) and quantitative changes (intensity and frequency) are important.

My prodromes of hypomania/mania are:
1.
2.
3.
4.
5.
6.
7.
8.

My prodromes of depression are:
1.
2.
3.
4.
5.
6.
7.
8.

A signal in isolation is not in itself a cause for alarm, but **if more than two of these signals are presented repeatedly over the course of 2 or 3 days, it would be advisable to contact the clinician.** The pharmacological treatment can be reviewed and a series of behavioural guidelines can be adjusted in order to prevent these early signs from becoming symptoms with greater consequences. Just as physical symptoms may signal that a person may be coming down with the flu and would activate a **plan to counteract or deal with the consequences,** there are guidelines that can be useful when warning signs are detected in bipolar disorder. In addition, it is always advisable to have a trusted person available who knows us and the disease well.

Action Plan after the Detection of Prodromes

At the beginning of a hypomanic /manic phase

- Increase the hours of sleep.
- Limit the number of activities, assigning significant amounts of time to sleep and rest.
- Reduce environmental stimulation, restricting the number of stimuli.
- Control mental stimulation with controlled breathing, relaxation, mindfulness.
- Avoid the use of substances that can worsen the symptoms (e.g. alcohol, caffeinated beverages).
- Postpone all important decisions and new projects. Confer with another person to evaluate the risks they involve.

- Delay economic expenses. Purchases should be postponed, preferably until the symptoms are in remission and, if possible, consult with another trusted person about the delay. If there is a suspected risk of inappropriate expenses, have the person surrender bank cards or delegate control of money to another person.
- Contact the psychiatrist and follow any subsequent recommendations.

At the beginning of a depressive phase
- Adjust the hours of sleep (around 9 hours). In the case of hypersomnia, activities should be scheduled for the morning. Napping is discouraged to promote restful sleep at night.
- Increase the level of activity. Start with the most urgent and important tasks (e.g. personal hygiene) and, slowly and progressively, introduce activities that previously were very enjoyable. Involving other people can also be helpful.
- Set realistic goals that are within reach for the person to help reduce as much as possible feelings of inadequacy or incompetence. Break down specific activities into more accessible parts.
- Postpone important decisions.
- Remember that no one is to blame for depression, and depression is transient.
- Engage in physical exercise to feel more energetic.
- Avoid the use of alcohol and illegal substances.
- Contact the clinician and follow any subsequent recommendations.

3.2.3 Treatment of Bipolar Disorder and Therapeutic Adherence

Medications, taken correctly, are the best way to prevent relapses. With each relapse, the person's vulnerability to new episodes increases.

Fortunately, there are many effective treatments that, together with a series of behavioural guidelines, can allow a favourable course for the disease, thus facilitating better functioning in all areas.

In bipolar disorder it is necessary to distinguish **maintenance treatment** (mood stabilisers) from **acute phase treatment** (antipsychotics and, in some cases, antidepressants).

Mood Stabilisers

Mood stabilisers are medications that help to calm and smooth mood swings. They are used to avoid the occurrence of new episodes and, in the case of relapse, to minimise the severity of the symptoms as well as their duration. Patients need to take mood regulators over many years, in most cases for life.

➤ One of the most common mood stabilisers is lithium, which has also proven useful in the prevention of suicide. Lithium's therapeutic effects (like its toxic effects) are related to its concentration levels in the blood, the reason it is important to have regular blood tests to harness its positive effects and avoid the risk of intoxication. The most common side effects associated with lithium are changes in digestive rhythms, tremor, increased thirst, greater need to urinate and modest weight gain due to retention of liquids. Effects on kidneys and thyroid function are rare but must be checked with regular analysis. Those circumstances that favour marked changes in body water volume (e.g. sauna, low-sodium diet, diuretics) can alter blood lithium levels. Lithium (as well as other medications discussed in this section) can interact with other drugs; therefore, the physician should be consulted before incorporating a new medication.

➤ Anticonvulsants (antiepileptic or antiseizure drugs) can act as mood stabilisers. They include carbamazepine, oxcarbazepine, valproate and lamotrigine. The latter has properties that prevent depression.

Antipsychotics/Antimanic Drugs

In bipolar disorder, antipsychotics are used mainly to treat manic or hypomanic episodes. They are very effective at eliminating psychotic symptoms (delusions and hallucinations), agitation, irritability, acceleration and other symptoms of elated mood.

➤ Among classic antipsychotics, one of the most commonly prescribed is haloperidol. Clozapine is also useful in manic/hypomanic episodes. Newer antipsychotics include risperidone, olanzapine, quetiapine, aripiprazole, ziprasidone, paliperidone, cariprazine, lurasidone, and asenapine, which are often used for preventive purposes. Some antipsychotics, such as olanzapine and quetiapine, appear to be useful as mood stabilisers. The most common side effects of antipsychotics are weight gain, decreased blood pressure, sexual dysfunction and some muscle stiffness, but these vary widely from drug to drug.

Antidepressants

For patients with bipolar disorder, the use of antidepressants can increase the risk of a hypomanic/manic episode or even rapid cycling (presence of at least four episodes in a year). For this reason, caution must be exercised with their prescription and they must never be administered as a sole treatment, but rather in combination with mood stabilisers and always under the supervision of a psychiatrist. It is important to bear in mind that it usually takes antidepressants 2 to 4 weeks to improve mood. Side effects, however, can manifest at the beginning of treatment (e.g. nausea and effects on sexual functioning).

➤ Fluoxetine, fluvoxamine, paroxetine, sertraline, citalopram, escitalopram, venlafaxine, duloxetine and desvenlafaxine are among the most prescribed antidepressants. Other antidepressants include mirtazapine, trazodone, bupropion and vortioxetine.

Other Treatments

➤ **Benzodiazepines:** anxiolytics or hypnotics, always under medical supervision, can be useful when anxiety is elevated or insomnia is experienced. In any case, they are not used as the sole treatment of a manic episode.

➤ **Electroconvulsive therapy (ECT):** this is an effective and safe treatment that can be used in cases resistant to pharmacological treatment or in which a rapid therapeutic response is required. The most common side effects are headaches and memory impairment during treatment.

> **Alternative therapies:** these are treatments not approved by the scientific community and so not considered standard care, because they have not been scientifically tested to demonstrate their efficacy, safety and tolerance. The danger of alternative therapies depends on their intentionality: those who choose to replace conventional treatment face a high risk of relapse.

> **Psychological therapies:** although pharmacological treatment is essential for bipolar disorders, psychotherapy can also be beneficial, but should always be instituted as a complement to medication. Psychoeducation, family intervention and, to some extent, interpersonal and social rhythms therapy, and cognitive-behavioural therapy are those that have proved to be, so far, effective in bipolar disorder. They all allow the person to understand the illness more deeply and incorporate training strategies and resources to handle it better (promoting protective factors and reducing risk factors) and to face stressful situations, thus reducing the risk of relapse. Some studies have shown that a combined treatment of medication along with these types of psychological therapies improves the course of bipolar disorder, both short and long term.

Treatment Adherence

Although pharmacological treatment is essential in keeping the mood stable, more than 50% of people with bipolar disorder do not comply with their agreed-on plan of treatment. Poor adherence can involve abandoning the treatment, making errors in dosing (e.g. skipping doses, not adhering to the schedule for dosing) or even neglecting proactive factors such as maintaining a healthy lifestyle.

There are many reasons for poor treatment adherence: lack of awareness of the illness or denial, real or feared side effects, feeling that the mood is 'controlled' by drugs, missing periods of euphoria, prejudices about the medication by the individual or those around them, social stigma, forgetting the scheduled dose. Identifying these reasons is the first step in dealing with adherence. Although no medication is exempt from side effects, these should not be reasons for abandoning treatment because the consequences of doing so are usually worse than the cost of maintaining it. Consulting with the psychiatrist about discomfort and fears allows for ways to be found to mitigate side effects, or to assess the possibility of modifying the dose or changing the treatment if necessary. Jointly analysing the pros and cons that result from the interruption of medication is essential, as well as seeking strategies to avoid forgetting to take the medication (e.g. pill boxes, alarms). Some people argue that the medication does not matter, because they have relapsed even while taking it. However, although the possibility of suffering an episode will never disappear, this probability will be lower in patients who take the medication correctly, and if under these conditions a relapse is suffered, they will be less frequent and severe and of shorter duration.

Stopping Treatment is the Most Common Trigger of Relapses. Other consequences include hospitalisations, increased suicidal risk, cognitive deterioration, problems in social and occupational functioning and economic losses. Assuming the need for sustained treatment and acting accordingly will reduce the frequency and intensity of relapses, and eventually will mean greater autonomy and less medication, while preventing the disease from interfering with the decisions and lives of the patient and the people around them.

Pharmacological treatments are not 'drugs'; they do not create dependency, they do not change personality and they do not avoid experiencing emotions, but prevent these emotions from reaching pathological levels.

3.2.4 Regularity of Habits and a Healthy Lifestyle

Regular and healthy habits (hours of sleep, healthy eating, avoiding the consumption of certain substances), **stress management and staying active form the basis for good health**. In bipolar disorder, the regularity of habits together with medication adherence are crucial in the prevention of relapses. Enhancing regularity of habits will lead to a better prognosis, well-being and quality of life. Promoting a healthy lifestyle is essential to improving physical and mental health. The initial effort may be less if we transform certain behaviours into habits.

Sleeping Patterns

Lack of sleep can lead to feeling more irritable and tired and affect concentration; in addition, it may interfere with performance in other areas of health and functioning.

The following **sleep hygiene guidelines** can contribute to better rest:

- Use the bed only to sleep and not to eat, study, watch television, use the computer or other tasks that involve stimulation. You can read before falling asleep, as long as it is not related to academic or work issues.
- Avoid solving problems and planning activities while you are in bed.
- Maintain an environment that favours sleep: ventilate the room during the day, and at night maintain an adequate temperature. Avoid light and noise.
- Try to have dinner at least 2 hours before going to bed, avoiding heavy dinners (fatty dishes), and eat a moderate amount to avoid going to bed feeling hungry or overfull.
- Do not consume stimulants or substances that contain caffeine/theine after approximately 4 p.m.
- Do not consume chocolate, large amounts of sugar or excess liquids.
- Engage in regular physical exercise, preferably in the morning. If you exercise in the afternoon do it at least 3 hours before going to sleep to avoid being overstimulated, unless it is light exercise.
- Avoid prolonged naps (no more than 30 minutes).
- Keep a regular sleep schedule, always going to bed and getting up at a similar time.
- Turn off the television, computer and mobile phone 2 hours before going to sleep.
- Before bedtime, include the promotion of relaxation (deceleration activities) such as lowering the intensity of light, listening to quiet music, having a warm shower, drinking a glass of hot milk or an infusion of tea without theine.
- If you cannot fall asleep, remain in a comfortable position with your eyes closed. If this is not possible, get out of bed and relax somewhere else, returning to bed when you start feeling sleepy.

– Do not use luminous bedside table clocks to avoid controlling the passage of time or seeing how long it takes you to fall asleep, as this contributes to increasing anxiety.
– Do not have an argument before going to bed.

In bipolar disorder, **a disturbance in sleep patterns** can act as a **trigger** of an episode (e.g. a decrease in the hours of sleep can precipitate a manic episode) or as a **symptom** (e.g. during mania, one experiences a reduced need to sleep and sleeps fewer hours). Therefore, **regularity in sleep patterns** can be used as a preventive tool and not only as an aspect to be treated in case of relapse. Controlling sleep hours can also help to manage the disease.

Some considerations related to sleep patterns in bipolar disorder

– **Sleep 7 to 9 hours every day** and, as far as possible, adhere to a fixed bedtime. It is required to sleep through the night, rather than sleep 6 hours during the night and then take a 2-hour nap to add up to 8 hours.
– **Schedules should be maintained throughout the week**; avoiding getting up very late at weekends as this may affect the quality of sleep on subsequent days. If you are getting to sleep late, it is advisable to sleep 8 hours even if it means getting up later. A disruption of the schedule should be the exception and not the norm.
– It is better to **have a job that allows strict regularity of habits to be maintained**. Those that include constant shift changes or night shifts are not recommended.
– It is useful, if you have not slept well, to **take a short nap** (maximum 30 minutes) to compensate, as long as it does not interfere with the quantity and quality of the night's sleep.
– For people living with bipolar disorder it is absolutely **inadvisable to spend a sleepless night** (e.g. for study, work, going out), since it could precipitate an episode. It is better to organise tasks in advance, avoiding last-minute forays.
– Hypersomnia or excessive daytime sleepiness, typical of some depressive episodes, can be combated by a reduction in the hours of sleep and an increase in the number of daily activities. A way to counteract the onset of a hypomanic decompensation is to **ensure a good amount of sleep for several days.**
– In cases of insomnia, **the psychiatrist may prescribe hypnotics or anxiolytics** for a brief period. This prescription should always be under medical supervision. It is important to avoid self-medication.

Nutrition

A balanced diet provides the nutrients and energy necessary for the body to carry out day-to-day activities, maintain vital functions and move around in the environment. Energy is balanced between intake, 'energy in' (food calories taken into the body through food and drink) and 'energy out' (calories being used in the body for our daily activity requirements).

Developing healthy eating habits to reach an adequate energy balance is not as restrictive as many people think. The essential steps are based on introducing foods derived from nature – that is, foods that are minimally processed – and increasing the intake of vegetables, fruits, lean meats, vegetable protein, whole grains and limiting the consumption of prepackaged and processed foods. Healthy eating means eating varied

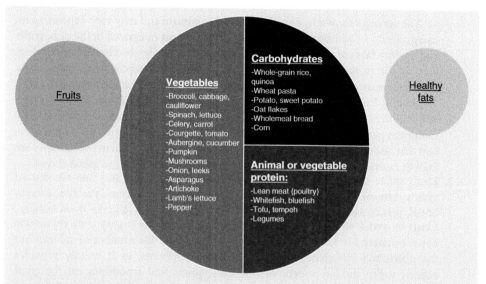

Carbohydrates
-Whole-grain rice,
quinoa
-Wheat pasta
-Potato, sweet potato
-Oat flakes
-Wholemeal bread
-Corn

Vegetables
-Broccoli, cabbage,
cauliflower
-Spinach, lettuce
-Celery, carrot
-Courgette, tomato
-Aubergine, cucumber
-Pumpkin
-Mushrooms
-Onion, leeks
-Asparagus
-Artichoke
-Lamb's lettuce
-Pepper

Animal or vegetable protein:
-Lean meat (poultry)
-Whitefish, bluefish
-Tofu, tempeh
-Legumes

Fruits

Healthy fats

Figure 3.2 Healthy distribution of food portions.

meals with portions appropriate to maintaining a good energy balance and a healthy mind. Nutrients protect health and prevent or delay certain diseases associated with unbalanced consumption and ageing itself.

Tips for healthy eating

1. **Control portion sizes.** We tend to overestimate how much we need to eat. Controlling portion sizes does not mean eating a little of everything, but rather choosing wisely what is put on the plate. Figure 3.2 is a suggestion of how to distribute food on a plate: half the plate consists of vegetables, one-quarter is carbohydrates, and one-quarter is protein, either vegetable or animal. A small amount of healthy fats and fruits rounds out the meal.

    Green, leafy vegetables should play a major role in a meal. Different varieties of vegetables, both raw and cooked, can be offered to add variety.

    Carbohydrates must be **complex** (not refined, but whole grain), because they provide the most nutrients. It is also important to alternate and try different options (e.g. quinoa, brown rice, potatoes, sweet potatoes, wholemeal bread, oatmeal flakes).

    Try to keep a balance between vegetable and animal **proteins**, prioritising vegetables whenever possible (e.g. legumes, tofu, tempeh, seitan, soy, peas, edamame). For animal proteins, choose the leanest meats (e.g. chicken and turkey without skin, lean beef, sirloin steak, pork loin). It is recommended to consume a minimum of three to four servings of fish per week and increase the frequency of oily fish (which contains healthy fats). Use low-fat cooking techniques (e.g. griddle, oven, en papillote, steam). Rather than using salt to add flavour to dishes, experiment with different herbs and spices (e.g. curry, rosemary, pepper, paprika, oregano, turmeric, nutmeg, cloves), so cooking also becomes an exercise in creativity.

The servings shown in Figure 3.2 are approximate and may vary depending on energy needs. In addition, although they do not appear integrated in the dish, **fruits and healthy fats** are no less important and are essential for good bodily functioning. Part of the portion size of the vegetables could be replaced with fruit. Fruit, preferably seasonal fruit, can be a between-meals snack (mid-morning or mid-afternoon). Examples of **healthy fats** include extra virgin olive oil, avocados, nuts or nut butters (e.g. tahini, natural peanut butter), Greek yogurt, dark chocolate (85% minimum purity), seeds (e.g. chia, sunflower, flaxseed), olives and eggs. It is important that healthy fats are present in meals but take care to limit them because they are high in calories. Use a tablespoon (equivalent to a portion size) to avoid excess.

2. **Limit sugar intake.** Try to limit eating white bread, pasta and non-wholemeal grains. Almost all precooked and processed foods (e.g. biscuits, pastries, cereals, bread, pizzas, sauces, sausages, snacks) have added sugars to make them tastier.

3. **Limit or avoid altogether sugary beverages.** A can of a sugary soda represents approximately 140 kcal. The problem is not so much the number of calories but the nutritional deficiency that this product represents, as it mainly provides refined sugar and no source of nutrients. Juices and smoothies can be good choices, but it is preferable to eat whole fruits because they provide fibre and satisfy more with a smaller amount. Coffee and tea are considered healthy drinks as long as they don't contain a lot of added sugar (or the amount of sugar is minimised as much as possible) and a high consumption pattern is avoided.

4. **Stay hydrated.** It is recommended that we drink between 1.5 and 2 litres of water per day. Make sure to have a bottle of water within reach and take small sips throughout the day, even if you do not feel thirsty.

5. **Apply the 80/20 rule.** Some experts talk about applying this rule for a flexible diet. It consists of healthy eating for 80% of the time and reserving 20% for treats (or not-so-healthy foods). Nutrition is not a matter of perfection but of finding a balance that can be maintained over time. This rule means that if you make a total of 21 meals a week (3 meals a day), you can reserve 3–4 'free' meals when you are with friends or family without having to worry about the food you consume during these social gatherings. At the end of the day, it is about doing what best suits your needs and lifestyle.

6. **Plan your meals.** Planning your meals in advance (the day before or making a weekly menu) can help you to better organise the shopping list and prevent you from eating unhealthily when you do not know what to eat due to tiredness or lack of time. A balanced diet should aim to nourish the body rather than counting calories. Moreover, not all sources of calories cause the same effect in the body. The way the body metabolises a doughnut as opposed to a chicken sandwich, for example, is completely different: varying hormonal and metabolic responses are generated that end up affecting the sensation of hunger and satiety after eating them. It's about choosing the foods we eat wisely, the more natural and less processed the better. If we are used to eating a lot of processed food, making this change will not be easy, but it is not impossible. Introducing changes in a gradual way could be the key to success. After all, the palate (and our brain) is educated. The appetite for unhealthy products will progressively diminish as soon as you start eating healthily and nourishing your body and mind.

7. **Sit at the table to eat and pay attention** to the sensations and feelings (hunger, if you feel it, taste, colours, smells, texture), as well as related emotions and thoughts.

Some Considerations Related to Nutrition in Bipolar Disorder

Changes in mood may involve changes in eating patterns. Hyperactivity, characteristic of manic phases, often leads to skipping meals; conversely, depression might involve either a reduction or an increase in intake. This, together with the potential effect of weight gain caused by some pharmacological treatments, reinforces the importance of healthy eating habits combined with a regular practice of physical exercise.

- Follow healthy and regular food pattern consumption. Excessively restrictive diets are not recommended, because they can increase anxiety levels.
- There are no 'forbidden' foods, the exception being for those who take monoamine oxidase inhibitors (MAOIs; antidepressants), who require a specific diet.
- Patients taking lithium should not abruptly initiate a low-sodium (low-salt) or asodic (no salt at all) diet, as it could interfere with blood lithium levels. Saunas involve an excess of sweating and could also modify lithium levels.
- A few studies suggest that intake of omega-3 fatty acids, in addition to pharmacological treatment, could contribute to improving mood stability.
- It is recommended that you discuss any alteration in eating patterns openly with your psychiatrist, including 'binge eating' (compulsively eating a large amount of food, usually carbohydrates, sweets or snacks, to calm anxiety or discomfort).
- Talk with your doctor about your fears of weight gain or possible side effects resulting from pharmacological treatment, in order to agree on the most appropriate treatment or to establish some guidelines to compensate for the side effects.

Physical Exercise

Moderate physical exercise represents a great benefit not only for physical health but also for psychological well-being. Therefore, performing moderate physical exercise periodically could decrease the risk of depressive relapse and improve well-being. It is also a way to reduce stress, and improve memory and sleep regulation. Physical exercise promotes changes in the brain that include neural growth, decrease in inflammation and release of endorphins, and increases the feeling of calm and well-being.

It is never too late to start building a stronger body and to benefit from the effects derived from physical exercise. Very few health problems preclude any kind of physical activity at all; if you have any problem, it is better to talk with a doctor in order to find a suitable routine. Physical exercise should not be considered a chore (no need to feel exhausted or stiff after every session at the gym) but rather part of a healthy lifestyle. Keeping a healthy body is a must since it can positively influence psychological health. You can build a strong body and mind with daily activities such as walking, swimming, cycling, caring for the garden or cleaning the house. Research shows that a moderate level of exercise is the best option.

But what does moderate mean?

- It means that you breathe with more effort than normal because of the energy you expended in the activity, but you do not run out of breath.
- It means that you feel warmer because of the energy you expended, but without becoming too hot or sweaty.

People who exercise regularly do so because exercise itself is a reward that brings more energy and better psychological well-being and promotes better mood, better sleep patterns and weight control. However, these are results observed over the long term. An exercise programme requires you to be disciplined and committed, which is not always easy. The following are some tricks that can help you to stay motivated and successful:

1. **Focus on activities you like.** Take some time to think about and explore the activities that are most motivating (or challenging) for you. The most important thing is to move, and any activity is valid: go for a walk with your pet, go shopping by bike, take an exercise class at the gym, take dance classes, hike, practise yoga, take a spinning class. If you have never exercised before, don't worry if you don't find a motivating activity the first time; keep exploring, and allow it to be an opportunity to deepen self-knowledge.

2. **Use the exercise as a social activity.** Exercising with your loved ones (partner, friends, children) is not only more fun, it is also a way to strengthen ties and build quality time, sharing experiences with the people close to you. If one is committed to someone, it can also make it easier to establish a new habit.

3. **Schedule it in your day.** Find the time to practise physical exercise. Even the busiest person can find some free time. Exercise should be a priority in your agenda: it is an appointment with yourself to build health. You can schedule it for early in the morning, during lunch break or divide it into 15- to 20-minute sessions throughout the day. Small sessions can be very effective in making your time well structured. If you are too busy during the week, you can concentrate on physical activity at weekends.

4. **Think about the reward.** Some days we don't feel like exercising because we are too busy, tired or cranky. However, keeping up the exercise routine during challenging periods is key to ensuring exercise's long-term physical and psychological benefits. A good strategy is to anticipate the positive emotion you will experience once the exercise is done: satisfaction with yourself because you overcame that mental barrier and the psychological well-being derived from the exercise session itself. On those days when you feel tired or are in a low mood, it is good to overcome these difficulties. Although it sounds counter-intuitive, exercising or participating in physical activities can give you more energy. If you are worried or overwhelmed, exercise can distract you from these thoughts and help you relax.

5. **Track your activity.** You can write down the days you exercise in a notebook. You can also add the type of exercise, duration and feelings/sensations. Tracking the activity increases commitment and helps you to monitor progress. It is also very motivating to review past annotations and check out your progress over time. Smartbands are useful here.

In addition to this commitment to physical activity, the following are some tips for an active life:

1. Walk whenever you can. Replace the car or public transport and bike or walk to work, to an appointment, shopping. If this is not possible, you can park farther away or get off the bus one or two stops before your destination.
2. Avoid lifts (elevators) whenever you can and use the stairs.
3. Increase your tasks at home or in the garden.
4. When you watch television, during advertisements take the opportunity to move or stretch, so it becomes a less sedentary activity.

Some considerations related to the practice of exercise in bipolar disorder

- Because of the stimulating effects of physical exercise, it **should be curtailed in the evening or at night** to avoid interfering with sleep quality or causing difficulties in falling asleep.
- In the case of an episode of **mania or hypomania**, physical activity must be drastically reduced. Exercise is stimulating and thus unadvisable during these phases. Never try to defeat mania through 'exhaustion' brought about by overactivity.
- During periods of depression, however, physical exercise can help us to feel better.
- During euthymia, exercise should be part of a normal routine.

Avoid Substance Abuse

When talking about psychological and physical health, it is essential to avoid drug abuse. By 'drugs', we mean all the legal or illegal substances with the capacity to provoke a physical and/or psychological alteration. They can modify the state of consciousness, behaviours, emotions and thoughts, and possess the capacity to generate tolerance and dependence in users.

Drugs are one of the most important risk factors in bipolar disorder because they can worsen the course and prognosis of the disease. It is likely that people with bipolar disorder who also present with drug abuse or dependence initiated their contact with drugs as a way of 'self-medication' before diagnosis. However, this type of consumption ends up aggravating the symptoms and creates an added problem that often requires treatment for both pathologies (bipolar disorder and addiction). On other occasions, some people do not present an addiction itself; however, even occasional drug use can cause relapses and worsen the evolution of the disease.

Selected drugs and their effects

- **Alcohol** is a central nervous system depressant. It causes depression in the medium term, increases anxiety, disrupts sleep, decreases impulse control, causes cognitive deterioration, increases aggressiveness and can cause psychotic symptoms.
- **Cannabis** can create an amotivational syndrome characterised by apathy and symptoms of depression; it can trigger a manic episode and sleep disturbances; it increases anxiety and can cause psychotic symptoms (i.e. paranoid delusions).

- **Cocaine** can trigger an episode of any kind, with rapid cycling, anxiety, aggressiveness, psychotic symptoms and sleep disturbances, and causes cognitive impairment.
- **Hallucinogens and designer drugs,** even if consumed only once, may lead to hospitalisation. They can cause psychotic symptoms that can persist over a long period and cause flash-back phenomena (repetition of symptoms weeks or months after consumption).
- **Tobacco** is harmful to health because it increases the risk of some types of cancer, affects the cardiovascular system and increases the risk of heart attack and stroke as well as respiratory diseases. Although it does not directly affect the course of bipolar disorder, interrupting its consumption has many benefits. A sudden attempt to quit tobacco can generate an increase in anxiety, so withdrawal should supervised. In bipolar disorder, drugs such as bupropion and varenicline, which are commonly used to facilitate smoking cessation, are not recommended. Because bupropion is an antidepressant, there is a risk of entering a hypomanic/manic phase or precipitating rapid cycling. Varenicline can also produce relapses. Quitting smoking is best begun in a period of stability (after some months of euthymia), with the help and supervision of a therapist, and through the use of replacement therapies (chewing gum or nicotine patches) to avoid the withdrawal syndrome that can lead to anxiety and irritability.
- **Stimulant substances** such as coffee can interfere with the hours of sleep and thus influence the course of bipolar disorder. Therefore, it is best to curtail coffee or tea consumption beginning in the afternoon. During hypomania or mania, it should be completely avoided. Other drinks that are strongly discouraged are the so-called energy drinks (e.g. Red Bull), which contain taurine, a stimulant.
- Benzodiazepines (e.g. alprazolam, diazepam, lorazepam) are the only medications that can create dependence if they are **misused or abused.** Therefore, it is important to follow a doctor's or psychiatrist's instructions. Never self-medicate.

Well-Being and Stress Management

An essential feature of a healthy lifestyle is managing stress (also discussed in more detail in other sessions).

Relatively mild, brief stress that remains under control can be stimulating, in a good way. Our performance can improve when we are slightly stressed. However, when we suffer stress that is too intense or sustained, the release of cortisol and a decrease in the immune response occur. In addition, stress can promote unhealthy behaviours. Stressors can be acute (sudden, sharp rise) or chronic (maintained over time). The body goes through three phases if the stressor remains: alarm phase (the body perceives the stressor and is predisposed to face it), resistance phase (maximum physiological activation trying to overcome the threat or adapt to it) and exhaustion phase (the organism exhausts its resources and loses its capacity for activation or adaptation). In this third phase it is likely that the most serious physical and psychological consequences arising from stress appear.

In bipolar disorder, stress can act as a relapse trigger in two ways:

- Directly: the physiological alteration causes changes in hormones and neurotransmitters that can cause a relapse.
- Indirectly: stress negatively affects sleep, and this may be the trigger for a relapse.

Although we tend to associate stressful situations with negative events, there are positive events that can also be stressful (e.g. a wedding, a promotion at work). It has been seen that the sign of the episode (mania, depression) does not necessarily correspond to the type of stressor.

Some of the stressful situations that we experience are a result of the duties and activities we carry out. However, **in stress management the interpretation of the situation, including the perception of the demands and the resources/skills we have to face it also play an important role.** Stress can affect physical, cognitive, emotional and behavioural levels. However, there are interpersonal differences in the response to stress, which makes some people perceive a situation as more stressful than would others.

Facing a stressful situation should involve **objective and rational thoughts, and a greater sense of control. Therefore, training in assertiveness, communication skills and the resolution of problems** can contribute to a greater perception of **self-efficacy** given a potentially stressful event. These techniques can also be part of an integrative programme that includes coping strategies centred on the problem and coping strategies focused on emotion. There are also strategies that contribute to **reducing mental and physiological** activation, as explained below.

One of the most commonly used techniques is **Jacobson's progressive muscle relaxation,** which consists of contraction and subsequent relaxation of each muscle, paying attention to the different sensations that occur throughout the exercise.

Controlled or diaphragmatic breathing consists of taking a deep breath in through the nose, inhaling it into the lower area of the lungs, pausing briefly and finally releasing it slowly through the mouth.

Mindfulness, defined as deliberately paying attention in the present moment without judging, and focusing on how the experience develops from moment to moment, can be useful training. It can be carried out by combining formal with informal practice (the latter to be incorporated in everyday situations), as will be explained in subsequent sessions.

The best action is **prevention of stress.** Often, the level of stress can be reduced with good **planning and establishing priorities,** in addition to incorporating into our day-to-day lives **rewarding moments and rest, physical exercise and a supportive social network that provides us with satisfactory relationships.** Dedicating time to the practice of these strategies is important.

During the session:
- Diaphragmatic breathing training.
- Explanation of Jacobson's progressive muscle relaxation (CD to practise at home).

Different apps are provided (related to physical exercise, nutrition, mood monitoring and regularity of habits) to help the participants delve deeper into the aspects worked on and discussed.

3.2.5 Psychoeducation Directed at Family Members: Family and Bipolar Disorder

Each episode of bipolar disorder is a stressful event for both the patient and those around him or her. It can alter family dynamics and generate fear and concern in all family members. Understanding what the disease is and having the resources to deal with it will improve the quality of life for all family members. **By accepting and understanding the disease, those affected and their families can contribute to the prevention of, detection of and coping with episodes, thus facilitating a better course of the disease.** The prevention of relapses will also avoid the negative consequences of the episodes (e.g. hospitalisations, problems in social or occupational functioning, risk situations, cognitive deficits). It is also **essential that family members pay attention and dedicate time to taking care of their own physical and mental health.** This session, delivered only to relatives or main caregivers, is part of an integrative approach to treating bipolar disorder.

Bipolar disorder is a **chronic** (lifelong) and **recurrent** (episodes tend to be repeated, although with appropriate treatment they can be avoided or reduced) illness, explained by an **alteration in the biological mechanisms that regulate mood,** located in a part of the brain called the limbic system.

People with bipolar disorder have mood changes characterised by periods of **hypomania or mania** (abnormally and persistently elevated, expansive or irritable mood and increased activity or energy) and periods of **depression** (feelings of sadness or despair, a loss of interest or pleasure in almost all activities). These phases alternate with periods of **stability (euthymia).** Both the intensity and frequency of these fluctuations will vary from person to person. **Early identification of the onset of new episodes will allow them to be dealt with as they appear and thus prevent relapses and their potential consequences.**

Bipolar disorder affects approximately **4%** of the general population and onset can occur at any time, although it is most often around the age of 20. Bipolar disorder is **not** an alteration of character or personality.

Bipolar disorder has a **biological basis and is genetically transmitted.** Individuals with bipolar disorder often have a relative who had or has similar forms of the illness, although it is also possible for subjects with no family history to manifest the disease. Biologically, it is important to note the importance of neurotransmitters (e.g. dopamine, serotonin, noradrenaline, acetylcholine), which are the substances that carry information through the brain. Neurotransmitters function abnormally during affective episodes; medication makes it possible to regulate these anomalies. Hormonal function, among others, also appears to play an important role in the disorder, as evidenced by mood swings that can be caused by changes in thyroid hormones.

Environmental factors are not the cause of bipolar disorder, but they may influence the course of the disease, either positively (factors that act as protectors) or negatively (factors that act as triggers for relapses).

➤ Main **triggers** include the following:

- **Discontinuing medication** or taking it incorrectly.
- **Irregularity of habits,** especially the reduction of hours of sleep. Anything that may negatively affect sleeping hours (e.g. afternoon/evening coffee consumption) should be avoided to ensure an average of 8 hours of sleep per day.

- Abuse of **drugs**.
- Stress.

Controlling, as far as possible, these factors, encouraging good therapeutic adherence, promoting the regularity of habits and a healthy lifestyle, and controlling the level of stress, among others, will contribute to reducing their negative impact on the course of the disease.

The **family environment** can act either as a protector or as a trigger for relapses. Bipolar illness can clearly affect family functioning; likewise, family functioning can influence the course of the illness. In the process of acceptance of the disorder, certain resistances can surface, which can lead to **denial** of the illness (e.g. attempts to explain the disorder as the personality of the patient, as a consequence of circumstances). Attributing voluntary control of symptoms to the patient can result in criticism, blame and conflict. At the opposite extreme, fear of relapses can lead to **overprotection and hypervigilance** that in turn can produce an interpretation of the patient's emotions, behaviours or reactions as if they were solely products of the illness – that is, seeing normal emotions or wishes as pathological. Although both positions may be understandable, in order to improve the course of the illness and one's own well-being, the **acceptance** of the disorder is fundamental, avoiding both denial and hypervigilance. The family must learn to **adjust expectations and behaviours** according to the phase of the illness, encouraging autonomy in times of stability.

Pharmacological treatment is essential for bipolar disorder. There are very effective treatments that, together with a series of behavioural guidelines, will contribute to improving the course of the illness and, as a consequence, family, social and work functioning, also increasing the quality of life. **Taking medication correctly is the best way to avoid relapses. The family's attitude towards the treatment can play a crucial role**. It is important for the family to develop an understanding of the situation that strengthens medication adherence, avoiding negative comments about medication and side effects. If the treatment is effective, some side effects should be tolerated, especially in cases where other medications have not worked. It is important to remember that the medication is not addictive, it doesn't produce dependency or tolerance, and it has been evaluated and tested very thoroughly so that the side effects have been determined not to harm the patient's health. Sometimes, fears and misconceptions about a treatment can manifest in negative attitudes and behaviours. If there are doubts about the treatment, the family should always consult the clinician. Medication should not become a subject of family conflict. **The level of involvement will vary depending on where the patient is in the course of the illness**. Greater control in the case of decompensation is understandable. However, if the person is stable, hypervigilant behaviours or excessive control can be counterproductive; in this case, if there is illness awareness, the patient should be responsible for taking the medication, and autonomy should be encouraged.

In bipolar disorder it is necessary to distinguish maintenance treatment (mood stabilisers) from the treatment of the acute phases of mania (antipsychotics) and depression (in severe cases, antidepressants can be used). Mood stabilisers help to even out mood swings. In general, people with bipolar disorder should take mood stabilisers throughout their lives to prevent further episodes, and in the event of a relapse, to reduce both severity and duration. The most commonly used mood stabilisers are lithium, carbamazepine, valproate and lamotrigine. The therapeutic effects of lithium (as well as its toxic effects) are related to its blood concentration levels, hence the importance of carrying out periodic blood analyses (lithaemias). Some antipsychotics, such as olanzapine and quetiapine, appear to be useful as mood stabilisers.

Psychotherapy can also be beneficial in bipolar disorder but should always be used as a **complement** to pharmacological treatment. Not all therapies are equally effective. Most of the effective psychological therapies for bipolar disorder, such as psychoeducation, allow the person to know the disease in greater depth and to learn coping strategies to manage the illness better, thus reducing the risk of relapses.

Acceptance and understanding of the disease and its management must be accompanied by caregivers' self-care, as it is essential that family members take care of themselves.

Some recommendations for family members

- Accept the illness and learn about it.
- Learn to detect the warning signs of possible relapses.
- Encourage good adherence to medication.
- Promote healthy and regular habits.
- Avoid blaming the patient or blaming oneself for the illness.
- Avoid criticism and overprotection. Promote a positive family atmosphere through good communication and problem solving. Learn how to find the right way and the right time to communicate and negotiate solutions.
- Be tolerant and adjust expectations and coping skills depending on the phase of the illness. For example, after an episode it is important to be patient because recovery will be gradual. In times of stability, encourage patient autonomy and empower each member of the family, including oneself, to have his or her own personal space and to assume different roles.
- Set realistic goals for yourself, and control the level of self-demand, being able to ask for/accept help, and assuming your own limitations. Accept that there are aspects that as a caregiver you cannot control.
- Learn to be assertive, giving space to your personal needs.
- Practise self-observation, attending to signs of fatigue or stress, and taking care of one's health, seeking help when necessary.
- Learn to relax through distractions, rewarding activities, controlled breathing, muscle relaxation and mindfulness. This will also allow you to better regulate emotions.
- Avoid isolation, strengthening your social network.

3.2.6 Mindfulness I: Automatic Pilot versus Awareness

What does our day-to-day life usually involve?

- **Running** to perform any activity without being attentive.
- **Eating quickly** (usually in excessive amounts) while watching television or talking, without paying attention to the process of eating itself.
- **Difficulty perceiving feelings,** physical tension or subtle discomfort.

- Thinking continuously about **past or future events**, without enjoying the present.
- Considering **thoughts as something true and real**, rather than as mental events that may or may not correspond to reality.
- Relating to experience through **thought** rather than directly experiencing it. This leads us to **judge** what happens to us as good or bad, pleasant or unpleasant and, consequently, to **attach** to the experiences that we judge as pleasant and wanting to **avoid or escape** from those that are unpleasant, instead of observing them and learning from them.
- Desiring things to be different from the way they are, instead of allowing them to be as they are.
- Being tough and critical with ourselves, instead of kind and compassionate.

Summarising:

➤ **We tend to live on 'autopilot'** instead of experiencing our lives in a conscious and deliberate way. Automatic pilot refers to the tendency to behave like automata, without focusing attention on or being aware of what is really happening from moment to moment. As a consequence, we can become ineffective in our tasks and not apply important information gained from experience, also affecting decision making.

Some examples:
- Missing a bus stop because we are thinking about what we are going to prepare for dinner.
- Eating a snack without paying attention to the smell, taste and texture.
- Taking a shower while reflecting on a work meeting we have to attend.
- Forgetting to take a medication because we are focused on a topic that worries us.
- Breaking things, having accidents or forgetting activities that we needed to perform because of carelessness or distraction.
- Driving without being aware of where we are.
- Avoiding a situation because of a past negative experience that we cannot stop thinking about.
- Criticising ourselves for having made a comment that is deemed inappropriate.
- Resorting to drugs or eating compulsively when we feel discomfort.
- Hearing someone but without listening carefully to what he or she says.

Mindfulness training allows us to be more aware of each moment, accept the experience and respond to situations with greater freedom of choice, without letting ourselves be carried away by automatic reactions.

Dr Jon Kabat-Zinn (1994, p. 4) defines mindfulness as:
awareness that arises through paying attention, on purpose, in the present moment, non-judgementally to the unfolding experience.

Mindfulness does not mean relaxation. Although sometimes mindfulness exercises can result in relaxation, it is not the goal of the practice. The practice is not oriented to achieve or 'get to' a certain state; each practice is valuable in itself.

Mindfulness does not mean leaving the mind blank, but observing what is happening in each moment, and when the mind wanders, bringing attention back to the here and now.

Throughout the day it is useful to ask ourselves, **Where is my mind now?**

Long-established mental patterns become habits. **Mindfulness training allows us to become aware of our mental modality.** Negative thoughts can provoke and maintain feelings of sadness. The training will allow us, for example, not to let ourselves be absorbed by rumination (allowing things to become a vicious cycle) that often contributes to accentuating feelings of sadness or personal ineffectiveness. In addition, being more aware of negative thoughts and moods will allow us to manage them better and have more control over their behaviour. **Paying attention** with an **attitude of curiosity and kindness** can reduce the reactions we all have to certain thoughts, sensations and emotions, which increases their duration and intensity. It allows us to **observe them objectively, as transitory events like clouds passing through the sky.** It increases, therefore, our ability to **accept and experience** sensations, thoughts and emotions without being trapped in them. This process makes us more aware of the alternatives that are presented to us, facilitating **less impulsive decision making.**

What does it mean to be in direct experience?

Being in direct experience means paying **attention** to the experience as it is, without expectation.

How can we get to observe our thoughts without 'hooking up' to them?

We can observe them **with curiosity, letting them arise and taking note** of them and what they promote ('pleasant', 'unpleasant', 'neutral'), as if we were an external and objective observer, a kind of scientist.

What is our goal?

Our goal is to embrace the experience, without getting attached to it or running away from it – **become aware.** Try to live the experience as if it were the first time, with the eyes of a beginner. **Leaving 'autopilot' allows us to be more aware and less reactive, which will improve our choices and decision making.** This approach simply allows the presence of physical sensations, thoughts and emotions that sometimes are difficult for us, adopting an attitude of **acceptance and kindness** towards them. It is not about resigning ourselves but accepting things as they are in the present and giving us time to choose the most skilful response to them. It is an alternative to avoiding unpleasant, difficult or painful thoughts, emotions and bodily sensations. We welcome whatever comes, **without judging.**

How can we achieve it?

Through practice, this is fundamental. We can distinguish two types of practice:

- **Formal practice.** Formal practice is that which is done in a regulated way, adopting a specific posture and reserving a specific time each day to perform it (e.g. with the help of an audio as a guide). To facilitate formal practice, look for a quiet place, have comfortable clothes and a light blanket if necessary, and reserve a fixed time each day to carry it out.

- **Informal practice.** Informal practice consists of performing our daily activities with full attention, which implies a different way of facing everyday experiences. For example, we brush our teeth paying attention to every movement, the sensation of water in the mouth, the taste of the toothpaste.

Both formal and informal practices are important. In both, the mind will tend to wander. It is then a matter of detecting that and redirecting attention to the present moment. Although this process always involves an effort, the more we practise the more skilful we will become.

We will enhance the practice both inside and outside the sessions. We will work together in the modification of mental patterns that were installed so long ago that they have ended up becoming habits. All new learning for change requires some effort, time and dedication. Therefore, it is essential for us to carry out daily exercises that allow us to learn about the habits of our mind and to modify them. The practice will allow us to be more aware of the present moment, detecting automatic responses and the tendency of the mind to wander and judge. If we observe carefully, the perceived experience can change. The difficulties that may arise (distractions, boredom, drowsiness, self-criticism) can be opportunities to observe, 'realise' and use in practice.

What benefits can the practice of mindfulness offer us?

Several studies point out the benefits of the repeated and regular practice of mindfulness on the reduction of anxious and depressive symptomatology, on the management of stress, emotional regulation, the ability to concentrate and, in general, on physical and mental well-being. In addition, we will be more aware of changes in our mood states, which can facilitate the detection of the first signs of alarm and the introduction of the most appropriate responses.

The Breath as an Anchor

Breathing has a special role in the practice of mindfulness; breathing is living. We can conceive of it as a thread or chain that links all the events of our life, from birth (the beginning) to death (the end).

- It is like an anchor that links us to the present moment, to the **here and now.**
- **It is always with us.** Most of the time we lose contact with our breathing but as much as we forget about it, it never stops being there, and it accompanies us 24 hours a day.
- **It does not produce attachment.**
- **It is changing and is linked to our emotional state.** There are no two equal breaths (there are always subtle variations in intensity, air characteristics ...) and it changes depending on our mood. Have you seen that when you are tense or angry, it is choppy and shallow, fast when you are excited, slow and full when you are happy, and seems almost absent when you are scared?
- It is a bridge **between the automatic and the voluntary.**
- In mindfulness you **do not have to manipulate** your breath, but just observe it.

Breathing Practice: Basic Aspects

- **Anchorage.** Breathe naturally, concentrating on the sensations associated with breathing: movement of the nostrils, differences in the temperature of the air entering and leaving, trajectory of the air through the body, changes in the thorax or abdomen when we breathe in and out. It is about observing our breathing with an attitude of curiosity.

- **Fundamental instruction.** To return to the notion of anchorage, when we have lost ourselves (if thoughts, emotions or physical sensations appear that distract us), sometimes it helps to briefly label the mental phenomena (e.g. thought, emotion, sensation, noise, or more specifically 'anticipation', 'comparison'). It is therefore useful to identify distractions and redirect our attention to breathing.
- **Attitude.** It is important to maintain a compassionate, caring attitude towards the mind and towards ourselves. The mind wanders continuously, and is like a restless animal. (Would we get angry with a small child who becomes distracted? Would we understand that a little dog moves from one side of the room to the other, continuously exploring the surroundings? Why don't we do the same with ourselves?)

It is irrelevant how many thoughts there are (the goal is not to have the mind blank). What is **relevant** are the following:

1. **The time it takes you to return:** we can't avoid leaving, but we try to return immediately.
2. **How we return:** it is key that it be with kindness, without criticising or getting angry, redirecting our attention again and again to the present moment.

Exercises to practise during the session:
- Eat a raisin with full attention.
- Pay attention to breathing.

Exercises to practise at home:
(It is recommended that participants use an audio – apps or links are offered to encourage the practice, as well as weekly practice logs.)
- Guided practice of attention to breathing.
- Mindful eating, at least once a day.

3.2.7 Mindfulness II: Habits of the Mind and the Importance of the Body

It is the nature of the mind **to wander** and we cannot prevent it from doing so. Therefore, how do we deal with that? It is worth emphasising that **mindfulness does not consist of 'emptying' the mind nor in avoiding the flow of thoughts, but in changing the relationship we establish with them**, without letting ourselves be dragged, overwhelmed or lost in them.

When the mind wanders, the goal is to identify it, realise where it has gone and then gently redirect attention to the breath, to the body or to what helps us to link to the present moment. **The essence of mindfulness consists of the willingness to start over and over, again and again.** Be more aware of the thoughts, emotions or physical sensations that you experience in each moment, as an external observer, to redirect your attention to the present, with a kind attitude. It's not about enjoying it; you just have to do it!

The generalisation of the practice: 3 minutes of breathing

Once you have practised breathing as outlined in the previous session, a generalisation exercise is necessary to apply what you are learning to a wide range of everyday situations. This exercise consists of three steps:

1. Detach from autopilot and become aware of the present moment by asking yourself, 'Where am I?' and 'What is my experience now?' Observe, without judging, your thoughts, emotions and bodily sensations.
2. Focus your attention on your breath, unifying the scattered thoughts in your mind to direct them towards an objective: breathing. Note the physical sensations and movements that accompany it.
3. Expand your attention to integrate your breathing and your whole body, being aware of your sensations, posture and facial expression. If you become aware of any feelings of discomfort, tension or resistance, focus on them, bringing the breath to that sensation with each inhalation and expelling it with each exhalation.

Allow and Accept

Situations are not inherently good or bad; it is our thoughts and our emotions that cause us to perceive them in one way or another.

We tend to seek pleasure and avoid pain. This tendency permanently stresses us as individuals, often leading us to insist on how things 'should be' instead of accepting what they are. Doing so creates frustration and causes us to worry and ruminate, without leading us to a solution and making us feel worse.

Each experience (i.e. each image, each sound, each smell, each flavour, each bodily sensation, each thought) automatically evokes in us a pleasant, unpleasant or neutral feeling.

- Our usual reaction to **pleasant feelings is attachment**: the need to cling to the experiences that have led us to them and to have more and more of these experiences.
- Our usual reaction to **unpleasant feelings is aversion**: the need to get rid of the experiences that have generated those feelings and do everything in our power to prevent them from repeating.
- Our usual reaction to **feelings that are neither pleasant nor unpleasant** (neutral) is **loss of interest**, boredom, disconnection and withdrawal from the experience of the moment.

When we resist and do not accept some pain, it increases, as reflected in the following equation:

Pain (inevitable) + resistance (avoidable) = suffering (primary pain + secondary pain)

For example, if we fall and break an arm, we will suffer an inevitable (primary) pain. If we also start to dwell on that and think, 'What bad luck I have, this sort of thing always happens to me', 'Why me?', 'How useless I am', 'This should not have happened to me', 'I'm clumsy', then our pain will increase, this suffering being secondary and avoidable. The crucial message here is that we can learn to free ourselves from the suffering created by ourselves.

The mindfulness-based approach allows us to 'be with' the problems without the need to **solve them immediately. The goal is not** to try to **control** the thoughts. The simplest way to **'let go'** is to stop trying to make things different. As a result, we will be less reactive and will be better at solving problems that require a solution.

What could we do, for example, when a strong emotion appears? A first step would be to acknowledge its presence, for example, before thinking, 'I'm tired of being talked to in that way' to realise, 'The emotion of anger is already here' and next, 'I'm afraid of the possibility of getting confused in that situation' to recognise and articulate, 'The emotion of fear is here'. Identifying and labelling emotions help us not to completely identify with them.

Accepting the experience simply means allowing space for what is happening. Being more aware of what is happening at each moment puts us in a more objective position from which to respond to difficult situations or negative moods, giving us the time and space necessary for decision making.

The Importance of the Body

We can train the mind using the body. Paying attention to the body provides us with another place from which to contemplate things, a different point of view from which to relate to thoughts and feelings.

Emotions have a bodily component. Sensations are an indicator of mood; therefore, paying attention to the body (e.g. where we notice tension, how the heart accelerates before an argument) gives us information about our emotional states and can help to better regulate emotions. In addition, paying attention to the sensations that we have not been aware of modifies our experience. For example, when we have many negative thoughts and emotions, paying attention to how these affect the body can give us a different perspective and change the nature of the experience. Bringing consciousness to the body can guide us when it comes to introducing aspects that can benefit us, for example intentionally modifying the posture or facial expression. If physical pain or discomfort arises, we must observe it with curiosity and openness, as well as the accompanying chain of associated thoughts and emotions. It may surprise us to discover how observing pain, instead of striving to avoid it, can change the perception of it.

Scanning the body will allow us to put these aspects into practice and also to train in the management of attention. The goal is not to make something happen but to observe what happens. It is about becoming aware of the different parts of the body, from the toes to the head, paying attention with curiosity to the weight, temperature, tension or any other physical sensation as it is presented in each body part, accepting the way we perceive it (pleasant, neutral or unpleasant), without any expectation, and redirecting attention to the body when the mind wanders. It is natural that the mind is distracted; what is important is being able to realise this as soon as possible and redirect it.

Exercises to practise during the session:
- Three minutes of breathing.
- Practise the dynamics of 'letting go' with pleasant, unpleasant and neutral experiences.
- Scan the body.

Exercises to practise at home:
(It is recommended that participants use an audio – apps or links are offered to encourage the practice, as well as weekly practice logs.)
- Perform a guided practice of breathing and scanning the body.
- Practise the 3 minutes of breathing at least once a day (you can use the mobile alarm as a reminder).
- Perform at least one activity each day (informal practice) with full attention. Examples: walking; brushing teeth; washing dishes; taking a shower; listening to music; drinking tea or coffee; eating.

3.2.8 Mindfulness III: Thoughts and Emotions

Thoughts

Thoughts are not facts, although we often take them as absolute truths, giving them a surprising power. Realising this is important, because **our thoughts (cognitions) greatly influence what we feel (emotions) and do (behaviour), and this interaction is reciprocal.**

What we are practising in these sessions allows us to be more aware of those thoughts that often tend to play a blocking or sabotaging role: 'This does not make any sense', 'I'm no good at this', 'Why bother if it will not work?'. This negative and hopeless internal dialogue is easily activated. In addition, it constitutes one of the most distinctive characteristics of depressive moods. If we let ourselves be carried away by it, we will not be able to counteract negative thoughts. From this derives the importance of recognising these thoughts and introducing strategies that contribute to breaking this vicious circle and consequently how we feel and how we act.

It is better to contemplate **thoughts as mental events and not as absolute realities.** We are often so closely trapped by them that we find it difficult to accept that they are simply partial and biased interpretations of reality. The thoughts or the ways of interpreting the events have a direct impact on our emotions and behaviour. In the same way, when our mood is low we tend to interpret things in a more negative manner, which intensifies discomfort.

There are different ways of working with thoughts. The **cognitive approach** consists of identifying them, being able to analyse the distortions of them and modifying their content. Since our emotions are influenced by our interpretation of the facts (and vice versa), a change of perspective can lead to an emotional change. The following list contains some of the most common automatic thoughts, because knowing what they are will allow us to recognise them when they appear:

- **Catastrophism** or tendency to expect catastrophes without reasonable grounds ('What if this headache is the first symptom of a terminal illness?').

- **Dichotomous reasoning** or perceiving reality in a polarised way (all or nothing, good or bad, success or failure, black or white), without nuances ('Everything goes wrong').
- **Overgeneralisation** or tendency to think that an isolated incident or event will happen again ('I will always be depressed').
- **Selective abstraction or mental filter**, focusing on a negative aspect instead of evaluating the situation as a whole ('Today I skipped the diet, I have no self-control').
- **Magnification of the negative** ('I made a mistake, it is terrible') and **disqualification of the positive** ('I passed the exam by pure luck').
- **Labelling** or, in the case of an error, adding negative qualifiers ('I am a disaster').
- **Emotional reasoning**, assuming that the way we feel is proof of the truth or reality ('I feel insignificant because I am so').
- **Arbitrary inference or jumping to conclusions.** Making hasty judgements without evidence to support them. Examples: 'mind reading' or making interpretations about the behaviour of the other, taking for granted what he or she thinks ('I am sure that he does not like me because we passed by and did not say hello'), the 'fortune teller error' or taking as true what we unrealistically predict ('It's not worth making an effort because I'm sure it will not turn out well').
- **The 'should' statements**, establishing rules that, if not met, generate guilt and discomfort ('I should like everyone').
- **Personalisation** or taking responsibility even without the foundation to do so ('My son has problems, therefore I am a bad mother').

From **mindfulness**, working with thoughts means being aware of their appearance but does not necessarily mean having to analyse or modify their content, simply 'letting go' without 'hooking onto' them. This approach can be very useful in the face of rumination or those unproductive thoughts related to the past (which we can no longer change) or the future (which has not yet arrived). Think of sitting by a stream and watching the flow of leaves floating on the surface of the water, or contemplating the sky and observing the passage of the clouds (which are transient). In that same way, mindfulness can help you to be more aware of the images and thoughts that arise in your mind without identifying with them and simply observing how they appear and vanish, if you allow them to do so. Mindfulness allows contemplation of mental events as if they were a transitory part of a whole. We can notice that thoughts and feelings give rise to bodily sensations and impulses that lead us to act in a certain way, and face them with an attitude of kind acceptance, choosing how to respond to them without being carried away by automatic responses or impulsivity. **Accepting that, for example, we feel sad or anxious** does not mean resignation, but it is simply a starting point that allows us to decide what we should do in a more skilful way. Sometimes it is not action, especially when it is impulsive, which is more convenient. Observing the experience in another way generates changes in it and puts us in a less reactive position for decision making.

Therefore, there is another way to relate to thoughts:

1. Observe with curiosity how they **appear and disappear**, similar to sounds, without letting ourselves be dragged along by them.
2. Consider that **thoughts are not facts** (they are not you, nor reality, nor the only possible truth) but mere mental phenomena.

3. **Taking note of the thoughts** allows us to consider them more objectively and, consequently, find them less overwhelming. In addition, the interval between having the thought and writing it or labelling it mentally ('This is the voice of depression', 'Here is the criticism again', 'This is a dichotomous thought') also gives us time to be able to respond in a different way.

4. Recognise the close relationship between thoughts, emotions and associated physical sensations, as well as the impulse to act, being aware that **our thoughts are only one link in a chain.**

5. It may be useful **to look at them again deliberately, from a more objective perspective based on evidence.**

Emotions

Emotions are a vehicular factor between perception and behaviour. A perception generates an emotion that will guide our action. The problem arises when we ignore the emotions or we allow ourselves to be invaded by them, leading us to act in a reactive or impulsive way. Being aware of the body's expression and behavioural responses related to emotions (fear, sadness, anger, joy) as well as to the function they have and the time in which associated thoughts are located could be an interesting exercise.

Since in bipolar disorder the emotions can become 'pathological', it is good to be able to apply full awareness to the emotion to recognise it when it arises, and to assess whether the associated behaviour is the most appropriate. We know that some behaviours can be more or less beneficial at certain points in the illness and therefore we will be able to introduce them if we are able to recognise certain emotional states in time to deal with them.

Emotional regulation, or the ability to handle emotions appropriately, is taught through becoming aware of the emotion and regulating our behaviour according to the context and requirements of the situation. First, we recognise the emotion by giving it a name (fear, anger, sadness, joy), accepting it without judging, noticing the impact it has on the body (e.g. breathing, muscular tension), noticing the impulse to react that it produces and being aware of the consequences that would result, and then being able to put it into perspective and decide on the most skilful response (e.g. paying attention to breathing or to other stimuli, cognitive restructuring, adopting certain behaviours). We can try to distance ourselves from emotion and become a compassionate observer (the metaphor of a mother holding her crying child can be useful). It is worth remembering that we are more than an emotion, that emotions can have an adaptive value and that they are changing and transitory.

In summary, mindfulness training (and that implies a lot of practice) can, among other things, make us more aware of our changes of state (mental, mood, body, etc.) and also of the first warning signs of a possible relapse, to allow us to recognise stress more quickly and to look for strategies to better manage it, to facilitate greater emotional regulation and strategies for the reduction of anxiety, to train our capacity of attention and concentration, to be more compassionate with ourselves, to improve our responses (so that they are less automatic) and decision making, to enjoy the present moment more and to increase our well-being.

Exercises to practise during the session:
- Pay full attention to sounds and thoughts.
- Reflect on the effect on the body and behavioural manifestation of the emotion, its function and whether the emotional triggers refer to the past, present or future.
- Pay full attention to emotions.

Exercises to practise at home:
(It is recommended that participants use an audio – apps or links are offered to encourage the practice, as well as weekly practice logs.)
- Perform a guided practice of the exercises worked on (attention to breathing, body scan, attention to sounds and thoughts, attention to the present, attention to emotions).
- Practise the 3 minutes of breathing at least once a day (you can use the mobile alarm as a reminder).
- Perform at least one activity each day (informal practice) with full attention.
  Examples: walking; brushing teeth; washing dishes; taking a shower; listening to music; drinking tea or coffee; eating.
- Resources are offered (links, apps and bibliography) to further deepen the practice.

3.2.9 Cognitive and Functional Enhancement: Attention and Memory

Cognitive functions are all those mental processes related to the acts of thinking, decision making, planning, remembering, paying attention, and so on. The importance of our cognitive functions lies in the role they exert in daily functioning: in our work or academic performance, in how we act in social interactions and in our environment.

Patients with bipolar disorder may have difficulties in certain cognitive functions, the most frequent complaints being those related to memory and concentration difficulties. Deficits are usually more evident during episodes of mania and depression, but in some cases deficits persist in clinical remission, that is, when patients have practically no symptoms of the disease. These difficulties, known as cognitive deficits, affect approximately 30–60% of patients with bipolar disorder, to a greater or lesser extent. Therefore, there is great variability and **not all individuals** diagnosed with bipolar disorder will exhibit cognitive deficits.

The most common difficulties exhibited by patients with bipolar disorder are related to attention, memory and executive functions.

1. **Attention** is a set of processes that allows us to be oriented towards a certain stimulus or situation and to ignore the rest. Its functioning would be similar to the spotlighting system, trained on one actor, in a theatre. Attention deficits manifest in difficulties in the capacity to select information in a clear and precise way, as well as maintaining it in our mind. Attention is the basis of the rest of the cognitive processes; therefore, the functioning of other cognitive processes may be conditioned by attention functioning.

2. **Memory** is a set of processes involved in the acquisition, storage and retrieval of information such as remembering past experiences, recognising information that was

previously learned, implicit learning (e.g. cycling or swimming), general acquired knowledge (e.g. capitals of European countries) or remembering things that we have to do in the future.

3. **Executive functions** refers to a set of complex cognitive functions needed to organise and plan, guide, review, regulate and evaluate our responses or behaviours in order to adapt effectively to our environment and achieve goals. They will allow us to anticipate unforeseen events or difficulties that may arise, to be less impulsive, to make appropriate decisions, to be flexible, to manage our time effectively and to adapt to new situations.

The importance of cognitive dysfunctions lies mainly in the fact that they can affect **daily functioning** on a personal, social, family or work level. For example, problems of concentration and attention may entail difficulties in maintaining a conversation with friends which, consequently, may result in social isolation. Difficulties in properly organising and managing our time may lead to problems in keeping up and finishing our work as quickly as necessary which, over time, can lead to complaints from our boss or even that we are demoted to a job involving simpler tasks. Difficulties in the ability to divide our attention will lead to problems in answering our partner's questions when we are doing another task at the same time (e.g. watching television), which will lead to tension.

There are different approaches to coping with cognitive deficits. **Cognitive or functional remediation** is an intervention that aims at improving cognitive functioning through training impaired functions or by the implementation of compensatory strategies.

In addition, we should bear in mind the cognitive decline associated with normal ageing, so training cognitive functions will always be a healthy way to contribute to mitigating this decline. The concept of '**cognitive reserve**' was proposed to refer to the capacity of the brain to cope with damage associated with specific neurological diseases or with ageing, being able to minimise and counteract this decline. People with greater cognitive reserve may have a delay in symptoms of cognitive decline in comparison with those who have a lower cognitive reserve. One way to increase and enrich cognitive reserve is by exercising the brain over the life course through an accumulation of educational and formative studies, engaging in intellectual and cultural activities (e.g. reading, learning a new language, playing a musical instrument), and participating in sports and leisure activities.

1. Attention

Some useful guidelines that may help to improve our attention capacity include the following:

a. **Reduce external distractions** to let you focus on what is important to you.

b. **Commit to paying attention** for a period of time (e.g. 20 minutes). You can use a clock or an alarm.

c. **Give yourself a reasonable and realistic amount of time** to complete an activity. This may mean modifying some of your expectations.

d. **Redirect your attention**, going from a more **global view** to the **most specific and relevant details** when you observe places or people. The **formulation of mental questions** about what you are observing may be a useful resource to use to redirect your attention.

e. **Plan rest periods (breaks)** during an activity (e.g. 5–10 minutes of rest every 20–30 minutes of activity).

f. **Change tasks at certain pre-established times** to avoid monotony and boredom.

g. **Take notes.**

h. **Establish routines** to avoid situations that involve more than one simultaneous task.

i. Use **'self-instructions'** to redirect your attention when faced with a task. This resource is based on the use of internal language as a behaviour mediator, allowing us to regulate our activity or, in this case, focus our attention. For example, before starting an activity you can ask yourself, 'What do I have to do?'; while you are engaged in the task, you will look for external clues to detect whether you have been distracted and thinking of something else: 'Am I paying attention to what I am doing?', 'I have lost my train of thought . . . I am going to focus again on what I was doing'.

j. **Reflective listening**: try to participate in conversations with reflective listening, for example, asking questions to clarify doubts or to confirm data. This will help you to focus your attention and, consequently, better retain the information.

Tasks to train attentional capacity include word searches, Sudoku, 'spot the difference', crossword puzzles, mental calculation (e.g. calculating change owed for a purchase when shopping) and other hobbies such as online games. There are several online cognitive training programmes available, including mobile applications, some of which have been shown to activate and strengthen cognitive abilities through the enhancement of brain functioning. Board games are also useful and fun.

Moreover, as has been covered in previous sessions, the practice of mindfulness techniques may be useful in making you better at focusing your attention on what you are doing or experiencing in the present moment.

Reading is a habit that enhances attention and concentration. For people who have lost the reading habit and would like to resume it or for those who have never been enthusiastic readers, start reading gradually. For instance, start with simple works and read for short periods at different times under optimal conditions (e.g. when well rested). As practice progresses, you will be able to spend longer periods of time and choose more complex readings.

The **'three-step method of reading'** will be useful to facilitate reading comprehension and the acquisition of information:

1. **First, read** without underlining or taking notes.

2. Go back and **underline** the most important aspects (ask yourself what has happened, where, when, how, who is involved and why; this will help you detect the most relevant information).

3. **Review**, reading the information that has just been underlined.

This method may be useful for reading short texts, news articles, magazine articles or readings related to an academic/educational or work context.

2. Memory

Some authors have compared the way memory processes work with the functioning of a library, which can hold thousands of units of information, in which memories must be well classified and coded to retrieve them easily (Figure 3.3). At the librarian's desk,

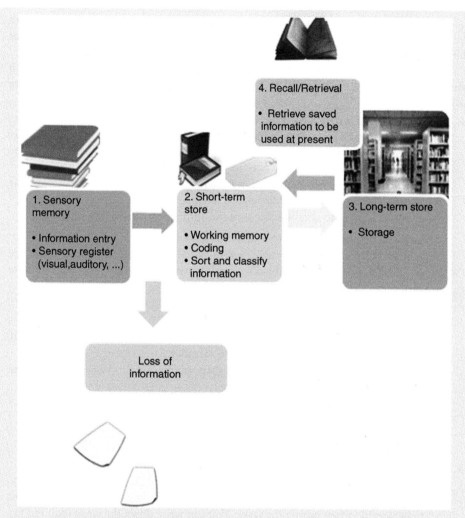

Figure 3.3 The library metaphor illustrates memory functioning.

the data to be stored arrive (**short-term memory**), so it is very important to label and code them correctly to access them easily (**coding process**). At that moment, perhaps some papers or books are lost or discarded (**information that is lost or rejected in the short-term memory**). Books already stored and well coded on the shelves (**long-term memory**) may also arrive on the desk when it is necessary to retrieve certain information (**memory or stored information**). Well-classified and stored data will be easier to recover. However, sometimes books or documents are badly classified or mis-shelved in the library, which makes access to them difficult (data or memories that we have but cannot retrieve). Memory functioning has also been compared to the functioning of a computer.

There are both internal and external strategies that can help us to remember things in our daily lives. Everyone should evaluate which strategies and techniques work best for him or her.

External aids are resources that offer many advantages since training is much simpler than that required by other memorisation strategies, such as those that are internal.

a. **Daily planner:** the use of a daily planner may help you to retain information about appointments, future plans or activities and important dates to remember. A planner can also work as a notebook, as it can contain a number of separate sections designed to respond to different issues (e.g. note sections, urgent items, monthly planning). Good use of the planner implies an activity and mental effort that can help increase the ability to code and retrieve the information later.

Important aspects to take into account for optimal management of the planner:

– Take the planner with you to note down what is necessary.
– Consult it daily. Review it every day at the same time to check what activities are outstanding. At the end of the day, check it again to plan the next day and note what is pending.
– Develop an easy notation system to allow quick access to information.
– Be concrete and concise when writing down tasks.
– Write down the most important appointments and activities of the day, even if you think you have committed them to memory.
– Devise a personal coding system to help you quickly visualise whether or not you have completed the tasks listed in the planner (e.g. cross out, underline with a highlighter or tick when the task has been completed) or their level of urgency (e.g. put an exclamation mark (!)).

Information that may be recorded:

– Data that can guide you on a personal, temporal and/or spatial level. For instance, write down a personal or important news event that happened that day.
– Tasks, appointments or activities to be carried out during the day. It is important to be specific when noting the tasks. You can write down the steps required to perform tasks or resources that are needed to complete them.
– Detailed lists of things or tasks (e.g. shopping list).
– Calendar. Many planners include an annual calendar. Crossing out the day that has ended helps temporal orientation.
– Birthdays of relatives and friends.
– Other data to be recorded are those relating to taking medication to keep track of therapeutic adherence, a simple registry of mood (with a numerical scale from 1 to 10) and hours of sleep per night. It helps detect changes in your usual pattern that could be 'warning signs' to consider in case of an eventual relapse.

b. **Computers and mobile devices:** these devices have programmes or applications comparable to the planner and they are very useful for everyday organisation. In addition, they incorporate alarm systems that may be programmed to alert you when an activity is scheduled and also allow you to repeat an alarm periodically.

c. **Alarms:** they are useful to remind you of non-immediate activities to do, for example taking medication, going to a meeting or attending a medical appointment, or as a timer (e.g. when baking something in the oven).

d. **Weekly or monthly calendar:** it is very useful to have a calendar in a very visible place in the house to write down appointments or important dates to avoid forgetting them and to be able to plan the week or month in advance.

e. **Lists:** apart from paper and pencil lists, new technologies allow you to use the note system to create lists, and some applications have even been developed specifically for it.

f. **Sticky notes:** these are coloured note pads with a self-adhesive backing. Writing on these notes and putting them in visible places (mirror, wall, diary) can be useful as a reminder that you have to do a specific activity, such as call the dentist or buy batteries. It will be important to date them and throw them away once the task has been completed to avoid confusion. It is not recommended that these be used as the only reminder system or as a usual procedure since it will be easy to lose or accumulate them without their having been checked.

g. **Pillboxes:** these are useful not only to remember to take the medication properly, but also to check that it has been taken in case of doubt.

h. Other external strategies to use to remember certain outstanding activities may be to **ask someone you trust** to remind you to do something (doing so should be used for a specific occasion but not as a general rule) and the use of **symbolic reminders** such as moving a ring or your watch from one hand to the other.

i. **Personal diary:** this can help you remember things you have already done (significant events or experiences that have happened during the day) and can become part of your autobiography. As with the daily planner, the codification and retrieval of information are reinforced by writing down experiences in the personal diary. The use of certain social networks (e.g. Instagram, Facebook) may also be useful for storing and later retrieving information about events that were published previously. In addition, access to photographs, reading comments on details or anecdotes can help you remember a trip, an excursion, the name of a restaurant you liked, a celebration.

Internal strategies include mnemonic rules to carry out a better process of information encoding. They consist of organising or associating the new information, attempting to give it more profound meaning. Thus, information will acquire a structure with more significance, which will facilitate retrieval. The use of these strategies improves with repeated practice. There are several internal strategies, but the following focus on what may be more useful for daily functioning:

a. **Chunking:** our capacity to remember information in the short term is limited, being reduced to an average of around seven information units. Therefore, it may be useful to chunk or split the information into smaller and more manageable units when you have to remember a large amount of data (e.g. an ID or driver's licence number, telephone numbers).

b. **Association:** this strategy consists of linking new information with something that is already known, therefore connecting, joining or linking one element with another. For example, if you have to remember a list of words, you can look for phonetic associations (words that begin with the same letter or similar letters) or semantic associations (concepts that usually go together). The association can be useful to organise objects at home and find them easily: set a place for each object (medicines, documents, tools, keys, purse, glasses, etc.) and put them in places related to their use. Another strategy related to association is the **story-telling technique**, which consists of inventing a simple story using the information (words) to be memorised, giving it a certain meaning through the use of verbal mediators (links) that facilitate associations.

c. **Visual imagery:** using imagination to generate mental images that facilitate or enrich the association between concepts can greatly help us retain information (e.g. if you have to buy bread, eggs and milk, it may be useful to imagine a scene in which you are dipping bread in a fried egg that is served with a large glass of milk to remember this small shopping list).

d. **Categorisation:** this strategy consists of grouping the information into blocks according to a common characteristic. Identifying the common characteristic of the data provides a meaning and facilitates the storage of the information, which will make it easier to remember later. For example, it can be useful to make a shopping list in which items will be grouped according to a category (hygiene, dairy products, preserves, meat, fish, etc.); to pack a bag for a trip; or to organise the kitchen cabinets or the drawers of a wardrobe.

e. **Remembering names:** pay attention to the name of the person you wish to remember from the first contact and repeat his or her name several times during the conversation. In addition, it will be helpful to associate the name with the name of a relative/known person, or with the name of a famous person, or with some feature that characterises him or her. The name could be associated with mental images.

f. Other internal strategies are the use of **acronyms**, a mnemonic technique that consists of generating words, or pseudo words, as an abbreviation using the initials or first syllables of the key words to remember; the **technique of repetition**, which consists of mentally repeating the information to be retained, in which we are forced to focus on that information, increasing the possibility of memorising it; and the use of **rhythm and rhyming**, for example, adding a melody to the material to be remembered will facilitate the possibility of accessing the stored information (e.g. multiplication tables).

Practical exercise

Organise the following clothing in a closet using a strategy to help you with the categorisation technique:

Shoes	Jacket	Coat	Belt
Handkerchief	Blouse	Sweater	Sweatshirt
Anorak	Sneakers	Pyjamas	Boots
T-shirt	Skirt	Socks	Shoes

Are you able to remember all the elements after finishing the exercise? Organising the elements according to common characteristics should facilitate later recall.

Web and mobile apps are used to train cognitive functions and to practise different exercises – word search, Sudoku, crossword puzzles, mental calculation, looking for differences. Board games are also suggested.

3.2.10 Cognitive and Functional Enhancement: Executive Functions

Executive functions are the cognitive domains involved in the execution and regulation of behaviours directed towards specific objectives. Executive functions include the ability to plan and organise activities, cognitive flexibility, abstract reasoning (identifying relationships between ideas, reaching logical conclusions), the ability to inhibit behaviours by ignoring irrelevant information and controlling interferences, and estimating and managing time appropriately. Executive functions allow anticipation and goal setting, as well as self-regulation during the execution of tasks, optimising the ability to carry them out efficiently. These functions are linked to frontal lobes of the brain that act as an 'orchestra conductor' of the brain. The frontal lobes receive information from the other brain structures, integrating and coordinating the information effectively in order to carry out all those behaviours directed towards a goal or objective.

Therefore, executive functions are involved in the ability to solve problems in daily life (the next session will be devoted to problem-solving training). Executive functions are also involved in the formulation of action plans, the modification of strategies according to the priority of the plan and maintaining the order in a sequence of activities and distribution of efforts. They allow us to be cognitively flexible to adapt the behaviour according to the demands required by the task or environment.

What follows is a review of some of the aspects in which executive functions play a role and why they are essential for good day-to-day functioning.

1. Plan of Activities

Carrying out a complex task with a specific objective implies the following:
a. **Defining** the main task to be performed.
b. Determining the **necessary steps** to carry out the task.
c. Establishing the **order of execution of the steps** to be carried out.
d. **Implementing** the action plan.
e. **Monitoring** the plan and introducing changes in case of unforeseen events.

The following are some general tips that may also be useful:
– Divide tasks into several steps or different components.
– Give yourself simple and clear instructions to help structure and progress properly in the task execution. Using internal strategies such as **self-instructions** helps self-regulation. As mentioned in the previous session, self-instructions help

to focus attention, but they are also helpful in inhibiting impulsive acts ('Think before you act', etc.) and promoting the achievement of objectives (stop: 'What am I doing?'; define: 'What is the main objective?'; list: 'What steps do I need to take?'; learn: 'Do I know all the steps to follow?'; check: 'Am I doing everything I have planned to do?').

- Know and use available external resources that can facilitate the execution of the task (e.g. if you want to visit a place where you have not been before, it may be useful to consult a map in advance or use navigation applications such as Google Maps).

2. Time Management

A good estimation and management of time will be an essential requirement for programming and organising all kinds of activities. This concept refers to the ability to judge, in an appropriate way, the time needed to carry out different activities and to regulate behaviour according to time restriction. Therefore, it will be necessary to do the following:

- **Estimate time** needed to perform each task, taking into account not only the resources needed to carry them out but also the unforeseen events that may arise and force us to modify the planned order of activities.
- **Plan** tasks **in advance**. Establish and follow a temporary schedule, avoiding leaving tasks until the last minute since doing so contributes to the stress level.
- **Establish priorities**. Prioritise activities according to their level of urgency and the deadline. Discriminate between what is important in your life and what is not a priority. For this reason, it is advisable to draw up a list or an action plan establishing the priority level for each task.
- **Specify the order** of activities. In addition to the urgency, the order established to carry out tasks may be influenced by other factors, such as proximity, availability of resources or means of transport, using the same route already planned, among others.
- **Be flexible** and know how to introduce changes to the usual routine and make some adjustments to the distribution of activities whenever necessary. It is recommended that you have an **alternative plan** to ensure that you can complete the activity in case of unforeseen events.
- **Delegate responsibilities if the situation permits** and you feel overwhelmed. It may be useful to consider delegating the execution of some of the planned tasks to others.
- It is advisable to **plan short breaks between activities** to avoid unnecessary mental blocks or burdens.

The use of a record sheet such as the one here will be useful to plan the order of activities as well as managing time on any given day (or week).

Record sheet

Things to be done	Resources	Time required to do the activity	Urgency level	Order in which it should be done
Urgent business at bank	Opening and closing hours, transport, necessary documents, bank card, ID card	45 min (including travel and management)	++	1
. . .	. . .	. . .	. . .	. . .
. . .	. . .	. . .	. . .	. . .

Urgency level: ++ Urgent + Important – Not urgent

Practical exercise

Peter is an administrative assistant for three people at his office. At 4 p.m. he has to have a room ready for a meeting, which implies preparing the material for 10 attendees, setting up the computer and projector, receiving the catering company at 3 p.m. and supervising that everything is ready just half an hour before the meeting. In addition, first thing in the morning, at 9 a.m., the three bosses ask him to do several tasks at the same time. One boss asks him to make a restaurant booking for next Wednesday at 8 p.m. for four people. The second one asks him to make 10 copies of a series of documents for the afternoon meeting, and the third asks him to go to his office immediately to take some notes to write a letter that he will then have to type up, print, have signed by his boss and take to the post office to be sent priority to arrive by tomorrow morning at the latest.

Peter's work schedule is from 9 a.m. to 5 p.m. Please organise the tasks that Peter has to do in the office using the Record Sheet for the time management and planning activities and recommendations that have been previously discussed during the session, taking into account both time and resources needed to carry out each of the tasks.

Other exercises to practise the use of guidelines for planning activities and time management include the following:

– Plan a weekend in the mountains.
– Plan a trip.
– Organise a surprise birthday party or a barbecue with friends.

Haste makes us prioritise what is urgent, always resolving those issues first and pushing back what is actually important. That can be very stressful. Important issues should not be allowed to become urgent, as they will usually require a certain amount of time to be resolved. Urgency does not make an issue more important. It is fundamental to know how to differentiate between these two dimensions: **important/not important** (it is or it is not related to my objectives) and **urgent/not urgent** (it requires or does not require immediate attention). The Eisenhower matrix includes these two dimensions of planning and time management. It may be a useful tool to use to increase our productivity or make us more effective in our daily lives, especially at work.

Eisenhower matrix

	Urgent	Not Urgent
Important	**Do** Do it now	**Plan** Schedule a time to do it on calendar, decide when to do it
Not important	**Delegate** Who can do it for you?	**Don't do** Do it later or eliminate

The so-called **time thieves** are another aspect to bear in mind regarding time management. The phrase refers to certain behaviours, habits, people or things that make us waste time. Some of these are generated externally, but others are created by ourselves. The first step is to know what they are in order to detect which of them are present and avoid interfering with our daily lives. Common 'time thieves' include the following: (1) personal disorganisation; (2) having confusing or unclear goals that will lead to a need to expend more effort; (3) not making decisions; (4) not knowing how to say NO; (5) inability to delegate; (6) procrastination, especially postponing those tasks we do not like or that we find boring; (7) bad communication; (8) interruptions by other people; (9) certain meetings in which there is no explicit agenda or objectives; and (10) emails and the Internet, social networks (e.g. Facebook, Instagram) and instant messaging (e.g. WhatsApp, Telegram). We should look for strategies to use to avoid some of these time thieves. For example, we can mute the mobile phone when we are involved in an important task, and it is also highly recommended that you uninstall notifications of certain social networks or instant messaging applications since they constitute a significant source of interruptions. Concerning email, designate a moment during the day and fix a specific time limit to deal with reading and answering email.

3.2.11 Problem Solving Skills Training

One thing we all have in common is that we face problems, with different levels of difficulty, which need to be solved.

Day-to-day problems can increase our level of stress, especially when we feel blocked by a certain situation and tend to avoid making decisions, postponing the solution and increasing the anxiety generated by the problem. At other times, we may make impulsive decisions that often involve wrong solutions that may even make the problem worse.

It is important that the attitude and commitment be towards resolution. However, symptoms can also interfere with problem solving. That is why it is advisable not to make important decisions when symptoms of the illness are present, and it is better to wait for periods of mood stability that favour objectivity and freedom in decision making.

The way we interpret a given situation (insurmountable threat versus challenge) and perceive the resources we have to face it (feeling capable versus thinking that we do not have sufficient skills) conditions the emotional reactions and the way we face it.

Problem-solving skills training can strengthen our competence in selection of effective decision making, which can contribute to reducing the level of stress (and therefore its potential influence on relapses). In order to learn the technique, it is convenient to start with a problem that does not generate much difficulty, and then be able to generalise the process to more complex problems.

Problem-solving training consists of the following steps:

1. Defining the problem.

    It is essential to define the problem in a specific way, as this will allow us to clarify what the objective is that we want to achieve. A bad approach or an overly general or unspecific focus on the problem can make its resolution more difficult. For this reason, it is useful to describe the problem in detail, specifying who, what, where, when and how. The more objective the description is, the better.

2. Finding possible solutions.

    A richer result is produced when alternatives are many and varied, no matter how far-fetched or absurd they may seem! It is about encouraging what we call 'brainstorming'; in this step nobody is judging or evaluating suggested solutions yet. The more potential solutions we list, and the more diverse they are, the more likely it is that some of them may be adequate. However, we will carry out this analysis later. Here we have to be guided by the principles of quantity, variety and postponement of judgement.

3. Analysing the advantages and disadvantages of the possible solutions.

    The adequacy of each solution to solve the problem will be analysed, evaluating its consequences. It may be useful to use (a) the two-column technique, noting the pros and cons of each option, and then (b) scoring each solution according to the previous analysis, taking into account the probability that the solution will solve the problem, the time and effort required, the short- and long-term effects, the associated risks, and so on.

Solution 1

Advantages   *Disadvantages*

Solution 2

Advantages   *Disadvantages*

Solution 3

Advantages   *Disadvantages*

. . .

Score (0–10):

Solution 1:

Solution 2:

Solution 3:

. . .

4. Choosing the solution.

The aspects that dictate the choice of a certain solution will be related to the analysis of pros and cons as well as scores from step 3. Sometimes a combination of solutions can be useful.

5. Planning the implementation of the selected solution.

Once a solution has been chosen, its implementation will be planned, also fixing a time to test whether it will be effective or not. It is important to decide the way in which the solution's success will be assessed in order to anticipate possible difficulties that could arise when putting it into practice, with the hope of foreseeing how to confront these barriers.

6. Implementing the selected solution and commend efforts.

The last step is to put the selected solution into practice and take the time to evaluate the results. It is fundamental to commend the efforts that the solution's implementation has required. Value your accomplishments, no matter how small.

In the case that a solution is not effective in resolving conflict, it is important to go back to a previous step to find other possible solutions, following the same procedure.

3.2.12 Assertiveness and Communication Skills

Have you ever been in any of the following situations? You've been in a queue and someone pushes in but either you don't dare say anything or you overreact; a friend owes you money but you don't dare ask him for it; you think you deserve a salary increase but it's hard for you to ask your boss; somebody asks you for a favour and although it is not convenient for you, you give in because you're afraid to say no. These are just a few examples of unassertive responses to everyday situations.

Assertive behaviour is situated in the middle of a continuum that ranges from **passive** behaviour (the person does not defend his or her rights or express his or her feelings, systematically yielding to others) to **aggressive** behaviour (the person does not respect the rights or feelings of others and adopts a domineering and defensive attitude). There are people who 'endure' so much that at any given moment they may react aggressively to an insignificant detail. **Assertiveness** implies that we are capable of expressing and defending our rights, desires, needs or interests without systematically attacking or yielding to others. It therefore implies respect for the other and for oneself, which means greater satisfaction with oneself and those around us. At the level of communication, assertive behaviour translates into speaking in the first person ('I feel, I want, I think') and facilitates setting limits or being able to say no when necessary, without disrespecting the other person.

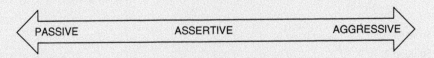

PASSIVE   ASSERTIVE   AGGRESSIVE

It will be easier to be assertive if we assume our **rights**:

The right to be treated with respect and dignity; the right to make mistakes and take responsibility for our mistakes; the right to make our needs as important as those of others; the right to change our mind; the right to ask for what we want; the right to reject petitions without feeling guilty, among others.

When the interlocutor is very insistent or manipulative, some **techniques** include the following:

- Viable agreement: give each person enough room to manoeuvre in order to arrive at a solution that is as convenient as possible for all parties.
- Broken record: repeat clearly your point, over and over again, staying calm.
- Fogging: agree with some parts of what the other person raises.
- Assertive postponement: useful when you don't know what to answer at that moment.

Mood affects the way we send messages and interpret the ones we receive, thus influencing communication. The existence of symptoms typical of depression, such as feelings of worthlessness or excessive self-criticism, or the lack of self-criticism and suspicion that can occur in manic episodes or when mixed symptoms are present, can introduce a distortion in the interpretation of messages received and affect the way the person expresses him- or herself. When a person's emotional levels interfere with interaction, it is advisable to stop the discussion and resume it when the emotional intensity has diminished. It is not a question of not talking about what concerns us, but of selecting the moment and the way in which we communicate.

Training in communication skills facilitates efficient and direct transmission and reception of thoughts, feelings and desires. It can therefore have an impact on problem solving and stress reduction.

Some **guidelines** can help improve interpersonal communication:

- Pay attention to both verbal and non-verbal communication; the latter includes facial expression, gaze, posture, and so on. Paralinguistic or modulating components (e.g. tone, volume, speed) also play a fundamental role.
- If symptoms from an episode are still present, it is preferable to postpone important decisions.
- If complaints or disagreements emerge, try being specific and do not generalise, focusing on the behaviour and not on the person ('It annoyed me that you didn't tidy the room', instead of 'You are an irresponsible person'). This makes it easier to find solutions and avoids the other person feeling attacked and therefore becoming defensive.
- Transmit clear and precise messages that cannot lead to misinterpretations (avoid vague terms, repeat the message, etc.).
- Listen well and pay attention, letting the other person express the message he or she wants to transmit without interruptions. Refrain from telling 'your story' when the other needs to express him- or herself.
- Don't invalidate what the other is feeling with 'that's nothing' comments.
- Avoid value judgements and attributions. Replace 'mind reading' with direct questions and avoid incorrect interpretations.
- Be flexible; keep your mind open to the ideas and suggestions of others.
- Focus on the present and speak in first person ('I need . . . ').
- Deal with one problem at a time. Raise problems as they arise, avoiding resentment and irony.

– Avoid distractions (e.g. tablet, mobile phone) as much as possible, as they can interfere with communication. Select an appropriate time and place for discussions.
– If there is an issue that is difficult to address, you can turn to a trusted person or a specialist.

Communication Skills

▷ **Active listening**
- Look at the person speaking and pay attention to what he or she is saying.
- Ask questions, clarify (avoid constant interruptions).
- Check that you have understood what you have heard.
– Summarise the message and ensure all is understood.

▷ **Expression of positive feelings**
- Look at the person and say exactly what you liked that he or she did.
- Express how that behaviour made you feel.

▷ **Expression of negative feelings and asking for changes**
- Look at the person and speak firmly.
- Say exactly what it was that bothered you.
– Avoid generalisations ('You always do the same thing').
– Focus on the specific behaviour and not on the person ('I was upset that you didn't warn me you'd be late' instead of 'You are irresponsible').
- Express how that behaviour made you feel.
- Indicate how to prevent repetition of the fact in the future.
– Suggest (speaking in the first person) what you would like the person to do ('I'd like you to let me know if you're going to be late'), instead of demand ('You should ... ').
- Express how it would make you feel ('That would reassure me').

To summarise: **describe** the behaviour that bothers you, **express** feelings in a positive way, **specify** the desired changes in behaviour and the **consequences** that they would have.

▷ **Refusing requests**
- Analyse the situation without rushing to make sure you have understood what the person is asking for, or ask for clarification or time to think about the answer if you need it.
- Look at the person and express your negative response in a friendly and clear way. Saying no is a right (if you want, you can give reasons, not excuses).
– You can directly say no, give a brief explanation or use techniques like the 'sandwich' (say something positive before and after refusing the request: 'Thanks for telling me, I can't help you today, but we can meet tomorrow'), or the 'broken record' if the other person insists after hearing your negative response (repeat 'I'm sorry but no' without having to justify your answer).

➤ Facing criticism

- Wait until the criticism is over before speaking.
- If necessary, ask for details to better understand the other's point of view.
- Assess whether there is something positive or constructive in the criticism.
- Apologise or agree if you believe that the criticism is totally or partially justified. If not, accept that the other person may have been bothered by a particular behaviour and explain your position without putting yourself on the defensive.

➤ Initiating, maintaining and finishing a conversation

- Take into account your and the other person's non-verbal language.
- Establish eye contact.
- Greet the person and introduce yourself, seeking the other person's attention.
- Introduce a topic to 'break the ice' or a comment on the situation or context in which the conversation is taking place (e.g. in a waiting room: 'Is there much of a delay? Have you visited Dr X before?').
- Ask for information, help, advice or opinions, paying attention.
- Share personal experiences, feelings or opinions.
- Show interest in the interlocutor with questions or praise (without seeming too eager). It is also important to be able to accept compliments if you receive them.
- With the intention of ending the conversation, express it politely and directly ('Excuse me, I have to leave') or even by making a small summary of what was said ('When we have more information we'll call each other then, okay?'), postpone the conversation for another time ('I would like to stay but now I'm in a hurry; is it okay for us to speak tomorrow?') or indirectly using non-verbal language (e.g. changing body orientation).

Although it is not always easy, it is beneficial to use an assertive response style in interpersonal relations, because it reduces stress in the social and family context, facilitates problem solving and contributes to increasing self-esteem and the sense of self-efficacy.

Appendix 1 The Group Rules (if the group format is used)

Over a period of 12 weeks, we will form a group that will meet every [*define a specific day and time slot that covers 90 minutes*]. From an integrative approach the aim is to contribute to a better understanding and acceptance of bipolar disorder, as well as to train in strategies to improve disease management, control stress and reduce the impact of the disorder.

In order to facilitate the optimal functioning of the group and to get the most out of your participation in these sessions, we have defined the following rules:

✓ **Respect.** All of the group's participants must respect the other members and their opinions, even when disagreeing. We don't allow demeaning, facetious or sarcastic comments towards others in the group. We can laugh together, but never laugh at another individual. It is essential to respect the others' turn to speak, listening to them and avoiding frequent interruptions.

✓ **Confidentiality.** A person's health condition constitutes part of his or her private life. The members of the group must be bound not to share private information outside of the members of the group. However, what we as therapists say and the material from each session can be openly discussed and shared with friends, relatives and acquaintances, as it is all general information related to bipolar disorder.

✓ **Attendance.** It is important to attend all programme sessions. Not doing so shows a lack of respect for those on the waiting list, and limits the understanding and benefit to be taken from the programme content. Any absence must be duly explained and justified. If absence occurs for more than three sessions, participants will be withdrawn from the programme, except in the case of a justified reason, in which case an assessment will be made for participation in subsequent groups.

✓ **Punctuality.** The group sessions take place on the same day of the week at the same time. It is important to respect the schedule; arriving late to the sessions interrupts their progress, affects everyone else in the group and prevents the person from taking full advantage of the programme.

✓ **Participation.** It is not compulsory to contribute in sessions, but it is advisable. We recommend active participation in sessions – answering questions, discussing doubts, sharing experiences – but all participants are free to choose the degree of disclosure and participation that they wish to show.

✓ **Distractors.** It is essential to keep your mobile phone silent during sessions.

In case of any doubts or problems you can contact the group therapists. Our contact details are the following [*names, emails, phone numbers*].

Appendix 2 Level of Satisfaction with the Intervention

We would like to know your opinion regarding the integrative approach in which you have participated.

☹ _____ ☺

0 1 2 3 4 5 6 7 8 9 10

Evaluation

Positive ☐   Neutral ☐   Negative ☐

Degree of satisfaction

Between 0 and 10, taking into account that 0 is not at all satisfied and 10 is very satisfied.

What contributions or positive aspects would you highlight?

Can you think of any suggestions or areas for improvement?

Bibliography

Aas, M., Henry, C., Andreassen, O. A., et al. 2016, 'The role of childhood trauma in bipolar disorders', *Int.J.Bipolar.Disord.*, vol. 4, no. 1, p. 2.

Altamura, A. C., Buoli, M., Caldiroli, A., et al. 2015, 'Misdiagnosis, duration of untreated illness (DUI) and outcome in bipolar patients with psychotic symptoms: a naturalistic study', *J.Affect.Disord.*, vol. 182, pp. 70–75.

Anaya, C., Torrent, C., Caballero, F. F., et al. 2016, 'Cognitive reserve in bipolar disorder: relation to cognition, psychosocial functioning and quality of life', *Acta Psychiatr.Scand.*, vol. 133, no. 5, pp. 386–398.

Baldessarini, R. J., Salvatore, P., Khalsa, H. M., et al. 2010, 'Morbidity in 303 first-episode bipolar I disorder patients', *Bipolar.Disord.*, vol. 12, no. 3, pp. 264–270.

Ball, J. R., Mitchell, P. B., Corry, J. C., et al. 2006, 'A randomized controlled trial of cognitive therapy for bipolar disorder: focus on long-term change', *J.Clin.Psychiatry*, vol. 67, no. 2, pp. 277–286.

Barbato, A., Vallarino, M., Rapisarda, F., et al. 2016, 'Do people with bipolar disorders have access to psychosocial treatments? A survey in Italy', *Int.J.Soc.Psychiatry*, vol. 62, no. 4, pp. 334–344.

Barnett, J. H., & Smoller, J. W. 2009, 'The genetics of bipolar disorder', *Neuroscience*, vol. 164, no. 1, pp. 331–343.

Baruch, E., Pistrang, N., & Barker, C. 2018, 'Psychological interventions for caregivers of people with bipolar disorder: a systematic review and meta-analysis', *J.Affect.Disord.*, vol. 236, pp. 187–198.

Bauer, I. E., Galvez, J. F., Hamilton, J. E., et al. 2016, 'Lifestyle interventions targeting dietary habits and exercise in bipolar disorder: a systematic review', *J.Psychiatr. Res.*, vol. 74, pp. 1–7.

Bauer, M. S., & McBride, L. 2003, *Structured Group Psychotherapy for Bipolar Disorder: The Life Goals Program*, 2nd ed. New York: Springer.

Bauer, M. S., McBride, L., Williford, W. O., et al. 2006, 'Collaborative care for bipolar disorder: Part II. Impact on clinical outcome, function, and costs', *Psychiatr.Serv.*, vol. 57, no. 7, pp. 937–945.

Berk, M., Post, R., Ratheesh, A., et al. 2017, 'Staging in bipolar disorder: from theoretical framework to clinical utility', *World Psychiatry*, vol. 16, no. 3, pp. 236–244.

Bojic, S., & Becerra, R. 2017, 'Mindfulness-based treatment for bipolar disorder: a systematic review of the literature', *Eur.J.Psychol.*, vol. 13, no. 3, pp. 573–598.

Bonnin, C. M., Sanchez-Moreno, J., Martinez-Aran, A., et al. 2012, 'Subthreshold symptoms in bipolar disorder: impact on neurocognition, quality of life and disability', *J.Affect.Disord.*, vol. 136, no. 3, pp. 650–659.

Bonnin, C. M., Torrent, C., Arango, C., et al. 2016, 'One-year follow-up of functional remediation in bipolar disorder: neurocognitive and functional outcome', *Br. J.Psychiatry*, vol. 208, pp. 87–93.

Bora, E., Bartholomeusz, C., & Pantelis, C. 2016, 'Meta-analysis of Theory of Mind (ToM) impairment in bipolar disorder', *Psychol. Med.*, vol. 46, no. 2, pp. 253–264.

Burdick, K. E., Russo, M., Frangou, S., et al. 2014, 'Empirical evidence for discrete neurocognitive subgroups in bipolar disorder: clinical implications', *Psychol.Med.*, vol. 44, no. 14, pp. 3083–3096.

Castle, D., White, C., Chamberlain, J., et al. 2010, 'Group-based psychosocial intervention for bipolar disorder: randomised controlled trial', *Br.J.Psychiatry*, vol. 196, no. 5, pp. 383–388.

Chadwick, P., Kaur, H., Swelam, M., Ross, S., & Ellett, L. 2011, 'Experience of mindfulness in people with bipolar disorder: a qualitative study', *Psychother.Res.*, vol. 21, no. 3, pp. 277–285.

Chatterton, M. L., Stockings, E., Berk, M., et al. 2017, 'Psychosocial therapies for the adjunctive treatment of bipolar disorder in adults: network meta-analysis', *Br.J. Psychiatry*, vol. 210, no. 5, pp. 333–341.

Chen, R., Zhu, X., Capitao, L. P., et al. 2018, 'Psychoeducation for psychiatric inpatients following remission of a manic episode in bipolar I disorder: a randomized controlled trial', *Bipolar.Disord.*, vol. 21, no. 1, pp. 76–85.

Chiang, K. J., Tsai, J. C., Liu, D., et al. 2017, 'Efficacy of cognitive-behavioral therapy in patients with bipolar disorder: a meta-analysis of randomized controlled trials', *PLoS.One.*, vol. 12, no. 5, p. e0176849.

Chu, C. S., Stubbs, B., Chen, T. Y., et al. 2018, 'The effectiveness of adjunct mindfulness-based intervention in treatment of bipolar disorder: a systematic review and meta-analysis', *J.Affect.Disord.*, vol. 225, pp. 234–245.

Colom, F., Reinares, M., Pacchiarotti, I., et al. 2010, 'Has number of previous episodes any effect on respones to group psychoeducation in bipolar patients?', *Acta Neuropsychiatrica*, vol. 22, pp. 50–53.

Colom, F., & Vieta, E. 2006, *Psychoeducation Manual for Bipolar Disorders*. Cambridge: Cambridge University Press.

Colom, F., Vieta, E., Martinez-Aran, A., et al. 2003, 'A randomized trial on the efficacy of group psychoeducation in the prophylaxis of recurrences in bipolar patients whose disease is in remission', *Arch.Gen.Psychiatry*, vol. 60, no. 4, pp. 402–407.

Colom, F., Vieta, E., Sanchez-Moreno, J., et al. 2009, 'Group psychoeducation for stabilised bipolar disorders: 5-year outcome of a randomised clinical trial', *Br.J.Psychiatry*, vol. 194, no. 3, pp. 260–265.

Crump, C., Sundquist, K., Winkleby, M. A., & Sundquist, J. 2013, 'Comorbidities and mortality in bipolar disorder: a Swedish national cohort study', *JAMA Psychiatry*, vol. 70, no. 9, pp. 931–939.

Daumit, G. L., Dickerson, F. B., Wang, N. Y., et al. 2013, 'A behavioral weight-loss intervention in persons with serious mental illness', *N.Engl.J.Med.*, vol. 368, no. 17, pp. 1594–1602.

De Rosa, C., Sampogna, G., Luciano, M., et al. 2017, 'Improving physical health of patients with severe mental disorders: a critical review of lifestyle psychosocial interventions', *Expert.Rev.Neurother.*, vol. 17, no. 7, pp. 667–681.

de Barros, P. K., de Ocosta, L. F., Silval, K. I., et al. 2013, 'Efficacy of psychoeducation on symptomatic and functional recovery in bipolar disorder', *Acta Psychiatr.Scand.*, vol. 127, no. 2, pp. 153–158.

Demant, K. M., Vinberg, M., Kessing, L. V., & Miskowiak, K. W. 2015, 'Effects of short-term cognitive remediation on cognitive dysfunction in partially or fully remitted individuals with bipolar disorder: results of a randomised controlled trial', *PLoS.One.*, vol. 10, no. 6, p. e0127955.

Depp, C. A., Ceglowski, J., Wang, V. C., et al. 2015, 'Augmenting psychoeducation with a mobile intervention for bipolar disorder: a randomized controlled trial', *J.Affect. Disord.*, vol. 174, pp. 23–30.

Fagiolini, A., Kupfer, D. J., Houck, P. R., Novick, D. M., & Frank, E. 2003, 'Obesity as a correlate of outcome in patients with bipolar I disorder', *Am.J.Psychiatry*, vol. 160, no. 1, pp. 112–117.

Faurholt-Jepsen, M., Bauer, M., & Kessing, L. V. 2018, 'Smartphone-based objective monitoring in bipolar disorder: status and considerations', *Int.J.Bipolar.Disord.*, vol. 6, no. 1, p. 6.

Faurholt-Jepsen, M., Frost, M., Ritz, C., et al. 2015, 'Daily electronic self-monitoring in bipolar disorder using smartphones – the MONARCA I trial: a randomized, placebo-controlled, single-blind, parallel group trial', *Psychol.Med.*, vol. 45, no. 13, pp. 2691–2704.

Faurholt-Jepsen, M., Vinberg, M., Frost, M., et al. 2014, 'Daily electronic monitoring of subjective and objective measures of illness activity in bipolar disorder using smartphones – the MONARCA II trial protocol: a randomized controlled single-blind parallel-group trial', *BMC. Psychiatry*, vol. 14, no. 1, p. 309.

Fiorillo, A., Del, V., Luciano, M., et al. 2014, 'Efficacy of psychoeducational family intervention for bipolar I disorder: a controlled, multicentric, real-world study', *J.Affect.Disord.*, vol. 172C, pp. 291–299.

Forcada, I., Mur, M., Mora, E., et al. 2014, 'The influence of cognitive reserve on psychosocial and neuropsychological functioning in bipolar disorder', *Eur.Neuropsychopharmacol.*, vol. 25, no. 2, pp. 214–222.

Frank, E., Kupfer, D. J., Thase, M. E., et al. 2005, 'Two-year outcomes for interpersonal and social rhythm therapy in individuals with bipolar I disorder', *Arch.Gen.Psychiatry*, vol. 62, no. 9, pp. 996–1004.

Frank, E., Soreca, I., Swartz, H. A., et al. 'The role of interpersonal and social rhythm therapy in improving occupational functioning in patients with bipolar I disorder', *Am.J. Psychiatry*, vol. 165, no. 12, pp. 1559–1565.

Gillhoff, K., Gaab, J., Emini, L., et al. 2010, 'Effects of a multimodal lifestyle intervention on body mass index in patients with bipolar disorder: a randomized controlled trial', *Prim.Care Companion. J.Clin.Psychiatry*, vol. 12, no. 5. pii: PCC.09m00906.

Gilman, S. E., Ni, M. Y., Dunn, E. C., et al. 2014, 'Contributions of the social environment to first-onset and recurrent mania', *Mol. Psychiatry*, vol. 20, no. 3, pp. 329–336.

Gliddon, E., Barnes, S. J., Murray, G., & Michalak, E. E. 2017, 'Online and mobile technologies for self-management in bipolar disorder: a systematic review', *Psychiatr. Rehabil.J.*, vol. 40, no. 3, pp. 309–319.

Goldstein, T. R., Fersch-Podrat, R. K., Rivera, M., et al. 2015, 'Dialectical behavior therapy for adolescents with bipolar disorder: results from a pilot randomized trial', *J.Child Adolesc. Psychopharmacol.*, vol. 25, no. 2, pp. 140–149.

Gonzalez, I. A., Echeburua, E., Liminana, J. M., & Gonzalez-Pinto, A. 2012, 'Psychoeducation and cognitive-behavioral therapy for patients with refractory bipolar disorder: a 5-year controlled clinical trial', *Eur.Psychiatry.*, vol. 29, no. 3, pp. 134–141.

Goodwin, G. M., Haddad, P. M., Ferrier, I. N., et al. 2016, 'Evidence-based guidelines for treating bipolar disorder: revised third edition recommendations from the British Association for Psychopharmacology', *J. Psychopharmacol.*, vol. 30, no. 6, pp. 495–553.

Grande, I., Berk, M., Birmaher, B., & Vieta, E. 2016, 'Bipolar disorder', *Lancet*. vol. 387, no. 10027, pp. 1561–1572.

Haffner, P., Quinlivan, E., Fiebig, J., et al. 2018, 'Improving functional outcome in bipolar disorder: a pilot study on metacognitive training', *Clin.Psychol.Psychother.*, vol. 25, no. 1, pp. 50–58.

Hayes, J. F., Miles, J., Walters, K., King, M., & Osborn, D. P. 2015, 'A systematic review and meta-analysis of premature mortality in bipolar affective disorder', *Acta Psychiatr. Scand.*, vol. 131, no. 6, pp. 417–425.

Hidalgo-Mazzei, D., Mateu, A., Reinares, M., et al. 2015, 'Internet-based psychological interventions for bipolar disorder: review of the present and insights into the future', *J. Affect.Disord.*, vol. 188, pp. 1–13.

Hidalgo-Mazzei, D., Mateu, A., Reinares, M., et al. 2016, 'Psychoeducation in bipolar disorder with a SIMPLe smartphone application: feasibility, acceptability and satisfaction', *J. Affect.Disord.*, vol. 200, pp. 58–66.

Hidalgo-Mazzei, D., Reinares, M., Mateu, A., et al. 2017, 'Is a SIMPLe smartphone application capable of improving biological rhythms in bipolar disorder?', *J.Affect. Disord.*, vol. 223, pp. 10–16.

Hidalgo-Mazzei, D., Reinares, M., Mateu, A., et al. 2018, 'OpenSIMPLe: a real-world implementation feasibility study of a smartphone-based psychoeducation programme for bipolar disorder', *J.Affect. Disord.*, vol. 241, pp. 436–445.

Hölzel, B. K., Lazar, S. W., Gard, T., et al. 2011, 'How does mindfulness meditation work? Proposing mechanisms of action from a conceptual and neural perspective', *Perspect.Psychol.Sci.*, vol. 6, no. 6, pp. 537–559.

Inder, M. L., Crowe, M. T., Luty, S. E., et al. 2015, 'Randomized, controlled trial of Interpersonal and Social Rhythm Therapy for young people with bipolar disorder', *Bipolar. Disord.*, vol. 17, no. 2, pp. 128–138.

Inder, M. L., Crowe, M. T., Moor, S., et al. 2017, 'Three-year follow-up after psychotherapy for young people with bipolar disorder', *Bipolar. Disord.* Abstract, DOI:10.1111/bdi.12582

Ives-Deliperi, V. L., Howells, F., Stein, D. J., Meintjes, E. M., & Horn, N. 2013, 'The effects of mindfulness-based cognitive therapy in patients with bipolar disorder: a controlled functional MRI investigation', *J.Affect. Disord.*, vol. 150, no. 3, pp. 1152–1157.

Jones, S. H., Smith, G., Mulligan, L. D., et al. 2015, 'Recovery-focused cognitive-behavioural therapy for recent-onset bipolar disorder: randomised controlled pilot trial', *Br.J.Psychiatry*, vol. 206, no. 1, pp. 58–66.

Kabat-Zinn, J. 1990, *Full Catastrophe Living: How to Cope with Stress, Pain and Illness Using Mindfulness Meditation*. London: Piatkus Books.

Kabat-Zinn, J. 1994, *Wherever You Go, There You Are: Mindfulness Meditation in Everyday Life*. New York: Hyperion Books.

Lai, J. S., Hiles, S., Bisquera, A., et al. 2014, 'A systematic review and meta-analysis of dietary patterns and depression in community-dwelling adults', *Am.J.Clin. Nutr.*, vol. 99, no. 1, pp. 181–197.

Lam, D. H., McCrone, P., Wright, K., & Kerr, N. 2005, 'Cost-effectiveness of relapse-prevention cognitive therapy for bipolar disorder: 30-month study', *Br.J. Psychiatry*, vol. 186, pp. 500–506.

Lam, D. H., Watkins, E. R., Hayward, P., et al. 2003, 'A randomized controlled study of cognitive therapy for relapse prevention for bipolar affective disorder: outcome of the first year', *Arch.Gen.Psychiatry*, vol. 60, no. 2, pp. 145–152.

Lazarus, R. S., & Folkman, S. 1984, *Stress, Appraisal and Coping*. New York: Springer.

Levin, J. B., Krivenko, A., Howland, M., Schlachet, R., & Sajatovic, M. 2016, 'Medication adherence in patients with bipolar disorder: a comprehensive review', *CNS Drugs*, vol. 30, no. 9, pp. 819–835.

Lewandowski, K. E., Sperry, S. H., Cohen, B. M., et al. 2017, 'Treatment to enhance cognition in bipolar disorder (TREC-BD): efficacy of a randomized controlled trial of cognitive remediation versus active control', *J.Clin. Psychiatry*, vol. 78, no. 9, pp. e1242–e1249.

Lex, C., Bazner, E., & Meyer, T. D. 2017, 'Does stress play a significant role in bipolar disorder? A meta-analysis', *J.Affect.Disord.*, vol. 208, pp. 298–308.

Lobban, F., Barrowclough, C., & Jones, S. 2003, 'A review of the role of illness models in severe mental illness', *Clin.Psychol.Rev.*, vol. 23, no. 2, pp. 171–196.

Lopez-Jaramillo, C., Lopera-Vasquez, J., Gallo, A., et al. 2010, 'Effects of recurrence on the cognitive performance of patients with bipolar I disorder: implications for relapse prevention and treatment adherence', *Bipolar.Disord.*, vol. 12, no. 5, pp. 557–567.

Lovas, D. A., & Schuman-Olivier, Z. 2018, 'Mindfulness-based cognitive therapy for bipolar disorder: a systematic review', *J. Affect.Disord.*, vol. 240, pp. 247–261.

MacDonald, L., Chapman, S., Syrett, M., Bowskill, R., & Horne, R. 2016, 'Improving medication adherence in bipolar disorder: a systematic review and meta-analysis of 30 years of intervention trials', *J.Affect.Disord.*, vol. 194, pp. 202–221.

Madigan, K., Egan, P., Brennan, D., et al. 2012, 'A randomised controlled trial of carer-focussed multi-family group psychoeducation in bipolar disorder', *Eur. Psychiatry*, vol. 27, no. 4, pp. 281–284.

Magalhaes, P. V., Dodd, S., Nierenberg, A. A., & Berk, M. 2012, 'Cumulative morbidity and prognostic staging of illness in the Systematic Treatment Enhancement Program for Bipolar Disorder (STEP-BD)', *Aust.N.Z.J. Psychiatry*, vol. 46, no. 11, pp. 1058–1067.

Martinez-Aran, A., Vieta, E., Reinares, M., et al. 2004, 'Cognitive function across manic or hypomanic, depressed, and euthymic states in bipolar disorder', *Am.J.Psychiatry*, vol. 161, no. 2, pp. 262–270.

Mellerup, E., Moller, G. L., & Koefoed, P. 2012, 'Genetics of complex diseases: variations on a theme', *Med.Hypotheses*, vol. 78, no. 6, pp. 732–734.

Melo, M. C., Daher, E. F., Albuquerque, S. G., & De, B., V., 2016, 'Exercise in bipolar patients: a systematic review', *J.Affect.Disord.*, vol. 198, pp. 32–38.

Merikangas, K. R., Jin, R., He, J. P., et al. 2011, 'Prevalence and correlates of bipolar spectrum disorder in the world mental health survey initiative', *Arch.Gen.Psychiatry*, vol. 68, no. 3, pp. 241–251.

Merikangas, K. R., Swendsen, J., Hickie, I. B., et al. 2018, 'Real-time mobile monitoring of the dynamic associations among motor activity, energy, mood, and sleep in adults with bipolar disorder', *JAMA Psychiatry*. Abstract, DOI:101001/ jamapsychiatry.2018.3456

Messer, T., Lammers, G., Muller-Siecheneder, F., Schmidt, R. F., & Latifi, S. 2017, 'Substance abuse in patients with bipolar disorder: a systematic review and meta-analysis', *Psychiatry Res.*, vol. 253, pp. 338–350.

Meyer, T. D., & Hautzinger, M. 2012, 'Cognitive behaviour therapy and supportive therapy for bipolar disorders: relapse rates for treatment period and 2-year follow-up', *Psychol.Med.*, vol. 42, no. 7, pp. 1429–1439.

Miklowitz, D. J., George, E. L., Richards, J. A., Simoneau, T. L., & Suddath, R. L. 2003, 'A randomized study of family-focused psychoeducation and pharmacotherapy in the outpatient management of bipolar disorder', *Arch.Gen.Psychiatry*, vol. 60, no. 9, pp. 904–912.

Miklowitz, D. J., & Goldstein, M. J. 2007, *Bipolar Disorder: A Family-Focused Treatment Approach*. New York: Guilford Press.

Miklowitz, D. J., Otto, M. W., Frank, E., et al. 2007, 'Psychosocial treatments for bipolar depression: a 1-year randomized trial from the Systematic Treatment Enhancement Program', *Arch.Gen.Psychiatry*, vol. 64, no. 4, pp. 419–426.

Miklowitz, D. J., Simoneau, T. L., George, E. L., et al. 2000, 'Family-focused treatment of bipolar disorder: 1-year effects of a psychoeducational program in conjunction with pharmacotherapy', *Biol.Psychiatry*, vol. 48, no. 6, pp. 582–592.

Miller, I. W., Keitner, G. I., Ryan, C. E., et al. 2008, 'Family treatment for bipolar disorder: family impairment by treatment interactions', *J.Clin.Psychiatry*, vol. 69, no. 5, pp. 732–740.

Miller, I. W., Solomon, D. A., Ryan, C. E., & Keitner, G. I. 2004, 'Does adjunctive family therapy enhance recovery from bipolar I mood episodes?', *J.Affect.Disord.*, vol. 82, no. 3, pp. 431–436.

Miskowiak, K. W., Burdick, K. E., Martinez-Aran, A., et al. 2018, 'Assessing and addressing cognitive impairment in bipolar disorder: the International Society for Bipolar Disorders Targeting Cognition Task Force recommendations for clinicians', *Bipolar.Disord.*, vol. 20, no. 3, pp. 184–194.

Mora, E., Portella, M. J., Forcada, I., Vieta, E., & Mur, M. 2016, 'A preliminary longitudinal study on the cognitive and functional outcome of bipolar excellent lithium responders', *Compr.Psychiatry*, vol. 71, pp. 25–32.

Moreno-Alcazar, A., Radua, J., Landin-Romero, R., et al. 2017, 'Eye movement desensitization and reprocessing therapy versus supportive therapy in affective relapse prevention in bipolar patients with a history of trauma: study protocol for a randomized controlled trial', *Trials*, vol. 18, no. 1, p. 160.

Moritz, S., & Woodward, T. S. 2007, 'Metacognitive training in schizophrenia: from basic research to knowledge translation and intervention', *Curr.Opin.Psychiatry*, vol. 20, no. 6, pp. 619–625.

Morriss, R., Lobban, F., Riste, L., et al. 2016, 'Clinical effectiveness and acceptability of structured group psychoeducation versus optimised unstructured peer support for patients with remitted bipolar disorder (PARADES): a pragmatic, multicentre, observer-blind, randomised controlled superiority trial', *Lancet Psychiatry*, vol. 3, no. 11, pp. 1029–1038.

Morton, E., Murray, G., Michalak, E. E., et al. 2018, 'Quality of life in bipolar disorder: towards a dynamic understanding', *Psychol. Med.*, vol. 48, no. 7, pp. 1111–1118.

Murray, C. J., Vos, T., Lozano, R., et al. 2012, 'Disability-adjusted life years (DALYs) for 291 diseases and injuries in 21 regions, 1990–2010: a systematic analysis for the Global Burden of Disease Study 2010', *Lancet*, vol. 380, no. 9859, pp. 2197–2223.

Murray, G., Leitan, N. D., Thomas, N., et al. 2017, 'Towards recovery-oriented psychosocial interventions for bipolar disorder: quality of life outcomes, stage-sensitive treatments, and mindfulness mechanisms', *Clin.Psychol.Rev.*, vol. 52, pp. 148–163.

Nierenberg, A. A., Hearing, C. M., Sande, M. I., Young, L. T., & Sylvia, L. G. 2015, 'Getting to wellness: the potential of the athletic model of marginal gains for the treatment of bipolar disorder', *Aust.N.Z.J.Psychiatry*, vol. 49, no. 12, pp. 1207–1214.

Nordentoft, M., Mortensen, P. B., & Pedersen, C. B. 2011, 'Absolute risk of suicide after first hospital contact in mental disorder', *Arch.Gen.Psychiatry*, vol. 68, no. 10, pp. 1058–1064.

Novo, P., Landin-Romero, R., Radua, J., et al. 2014, 'Eye movement desensitization and reprocessing therapy in subsyndromal bipolar patients with a history of traumatic events: a randomized, controlled pilot-study', *Psychiatry Res.*, vol. 219, no. 1, pp. 122–128.

Pacchiarotti, I., Bond, D. J., Baldessarini, R. J., et al. 2013, 'The International Society for Bipolar Disorders (ISBD) task force report on antidepressant use in bipolar disorders', *Am. J.Psychiatry*, vol. 170, no. 11, pp. 1249–1262.

Parikh, S. V., Zaretsky, A., Beaulieu, S., et al. 2012, 'A randomized controlled trial of psychoeducation or cognitive-behavioral therapy in bipolar disorder: a Canadian Network for Mood and Anxiety treatments (CANMAT) study [CME]', *J.Clin.Psychiatry*, vol. 73, no. 6, pp. 803–810.

Park, T., Reilly-Spong, M., & Gross, C. R. 2013, 'Mindfulness: a systematic review of instruments to measure an emergent patient-reported outcome (PRO)', *Qual.Life Res.*, vol. 22, no. 10, pp. 2639-2659.

Penadés, R., & Gastó, C. 2010, *El tratamiento de rehabilitación neurocognitiva en la esquizofrenia*. Barcelona: Herder Editorial.

Perich, T., Manicavasagar, V., Mitchell, P. B., Ball, J. R., & Hadzi-Pavlovic, D. 2013a, 'A randomized controlled trial of mindfulness-based cognitive therapy for bipolar disorder', *Acta Psychiatr.Scand.*, vol. 127, no. 5, pp. 333-343.

Perich, T., Manicavasagar, V., Mitchell, P. B., & Ball, J. R. 2013b, 'The association between meditation practice and treatment outcome in Mindfulness-based Cognitive Therapy for bipolar disorder', *Behav.Res.Ther.*, vol. 51, no. 7, pp. 338-343.

Perlick, D. A., Jackson, C., Grier, S., et al. 2018, 'Randomized trial comparing caregiver-only family-focused treatment to standard health education on the 6-month outcome of bipolar disorder', *Bipolar.Disord.*, vol. 20, no. 7, pp. 622-633.

Perlick, D. A., Miklowitz, D. J., Lopez, N., et al. 2010, 'Family-focused treatment for caregivers of patients with bipolar disorder', *Bipolar.Disord.*, vol. 12, no. 6, pp. 627-637.

Perry, A., Tarrier, N., Morriss, R., McCarthy, E., & Limb, K. 1999, 'Randomised controlled trial of efficacy of teaching patients with bipolar disorder to identify early symptoms of relapse and obtain treatment', *BMJ*, vol. 318, no. 7177, pp. 149-153.

Popovic, D., Reinares, M., Goikolea, J. M., et al. 2012, 'Polarity index of pharmacological agents used for maintenance treatment of bipolar disorder', *Eur.Neuropsychopharmacol.*, vol. 22, no. 5, pp. 339-346.

Rea, M. M., Tompson, M. C., Miklowitz, D. J., et al. 2003, 'Family-focused treatment versus individual treatment for bipolar disorder: results of a randomized clinical trial', *J. Consult. Clin.Psychol.*, vol. 71, no. 3, pp. 482-492.

Reinares, M., Bonnin, C. M., Hidalgo-Mazzei, D., et al. 2016, 'The role of family interventions in bipolar disorder: a systematic review', *Clin.Psychol.Rev.*, vol. 43, pp. 47-57.

Reinares, M., Colom, F., Sanchez-Moreno, J., et al. 2008, 'Impact of caregiver group psychoeducation on the course and outcome of bipolar patients in remission: a randomized controlled trial', *Bipolar. Disord.*, vol. 10, no. 4, pp. 511-519.

Reinares, M., González-Pinto, A., Crespo. J. M., et al. 2015, *Manual de psicoeduación para el trabajo con familiares de pacientes con trastorno bipolar*. Barcelona: J&C Ediciones Médicas.

Reinares, M., Papachristou, E., Harvey, P., et al. 2013, 'Towards a clinical staging for bipolar disorder: defining patient subtypes based on functional outcome', *J.Affect.Disord.*, vol. 144, no. 1-2, pp. 65-71.

Reinares, M., Sanchez-Moreno, J., & Fountoulakis, K. N. 2014, 'Psychosocial interventions in bipolar disorder: what, for whom, and when', *J.Affect.Disord.*, vol. 156, pp. 46-55.

Reinares, M., Vieta, E., Colom, F., et al. 2004, 'Impact of a psychoeducational family intervention on caregivers of stabilized bipolar patients', *Psychother.Psychosom.*, vol. 73, no. 5, pp. 312-319.

Rosa, A. R., Gonzalez-Ortega, I., Gonzalez-Pinto, A., et al. 2012, 'One-year psychosocial functioning in patients in the early vs. late stage of bipolar disorder', *Acta Psychiatr. Scand.*, vol. 125, no. 4, pp. 335-341.

Salagre, E., Dodd, S., Aedo, A., et al. 2018, 'Toward precision psychiatry in bipolar disorder: staging 2.0', *Front Psychiatry*, vol. 9, p. 641.

Samalin, L., Reinares, M., de Chazeron, I., et al. 2016, 'Course of residual symptoms according to the duration of euthymia in remitted bipolar patients', *Acta Psychiatr. Scand.*, vol. 134, no. 1, pp. 57-64.

Sanchez-Moreno, J., Bonnin, C. M., Gonzalez-Pinto, A., et al. 2018, 'Factors associated with poor functional outcome in bipolar disorder: sociodemographic, clinical, and neurocognitive variables', *Acta Psychiatr. Scand.*, vol. 138, no. 2, pp. 145-154.

Sanchez-Morla, E. M., Lopez-Villarreal, A., Jimenez-Lopez, E., et al. 2018, 'Impact of number of episodes on neurocognitive trajectory in bipolar disorder patients: a 5-year follow-up study', *Psychol.Med.*, Abstract, pp. 1-9. DOI:10.1017/ S0033291718001885

Scott, J., Colom, F., Popova, E., et al. 2009, 'Long-term mental health resource utilization and cost of care following group psychoeducation or unstructured group support for bipolar disorders: a cost-benefit analysis', *J.Clin. Psychiatry*, vol. 70, no. 3, pp. 378–386.

Scott, J., Paykel, E., Morriss, R., et al. 2006, 'Cognitive-behavioural therapy for severe and recurrent bipolar disorders: randomised controlled trial', *Br.J.Psychiatry*, vol. 188, pp. 313–320.

Segal, Z., Williams, M., & Teaslade, J. 2001, *Mindfulness-Based Cognitive Therapy for Depression*. New York: Guilford.

Selye, H. 1950, 'Stress and the general adaptation syndrome', *BMJ.*, vol. 1, no. 4667, pp. 1383–1392.

Shapiro, S. L., Carlson, L. E., Astin, J. A., & Freedman, B. 2006, 'Mechanisms of mindfulness', *J.Clin.Psychol.*, vol. 62, no. 3, pp. 373–386.

Simon, G. E., Ludman, E. J., Bauer, M. S., Unutzer, J., & Operskalski, B. 2006, 'Long-term effectiveness and cost of a systematic care program for bipolar disorder', *Arch.Gen. Psychiatry*, vol. 63, no. 5, pp. 500–508.

Simón, V. 2011, *Aprender a practicar mindfulness*. Madrid: Sello Editorial.

Sole, B., Bonnin, C. M., Jimenez, E., et al. 2018, 'Heterogeneity of functional outcomes in patients with bipolar disorder: a cluster-analytic approach', *Acta Psychiatr. Scand.*, vol. 137, no. 6, pp. 516–527.

Sole, B., Jimenez, E., Torrent, C., et al. 2016, 'Cognitive variability in bipolar II disorder: who is cognitively impaired and who is preserved?', *Bipolar.Disord.*, vol. 18, no. 3, pp. 288–299.

Starzer, M. S. K., Nordentoft, M., & Hjorthoj, C. 2018, 'Rates and predictors of conversion to schizophrenia or bipolar disorder following substance-induced psychosis', *Am.J. Psychiatry*, vol. 175, no. 4, pp. 343–350.

Stern, Y. 2009, 'Cognitive reserve', *Neuropsychologia*, vol. 47, no. 10, pp. 2015–2028.

Swartz, H. A., Rucci, P., Thase, M. E., et al. 2017, 'Psychotherapy alone and combined with medication as treatments for bipolar II depression: a randomized controlled trial', *J. Clin.Psychiatry.*, vol. 79, no. 2, pii: 16m11027

Sylvia, L. G., Friedman, E. S., Kocsis, J. H., et al. 2013, 'Association of exercise with quality of life and mood symptoms in a comparative effectiveness study of bipolar disorder', *J. Affect.Disord.*, vol. 151, no. 2, pp. 722–727.

Sylvia, L. G., Thase, M. E., Reilly-Harrington, N. A., et al. 2015, 'Psychotherapy use in bipolar disorder: association with functioning and illness severity', *Aust.N.Z.J. Psychiatry*, vol. 49, no. 5, pp. 453–461.

Torrent, C., Bonnin, C. M., Martinez-Aran, A., et al. 2013, 'Efficacy of functional remediation in bipolar disorder: a multicenter randomized controlled study', *Am.J.Psychiatry*, vol. 170, no. 8, pp. 852–859.

Torrent, C., Martinez-Aran, A., del Mar, B. C., et al. 2012, 'Long-term outcome of cognitive impairment in bipolar disorder', *J.Clin. Psychiatry*, vol. 73, no. 7, pp. e899–e905.

Torrent, C., Vieta, E., & Garcia-Garcia, M. 2008, 'Validation of the Barcelona Bipolar Eating Disorder Scale for bipolar patients with eating disturbances', *Psychopathology*, vol. 41, no. 6, pp. 379–387.

Van, D. S., Jeffrey, J., & Katz, M. R. 2013, 'A randomized, controlled, pilot study of dialectical behavior therapy skills in a psychoeducational group for individuals with bipolar disorder', *J.Affect.Disord.*, vol. 145, no. 3, pp. 386–393.

Vancampfort, D., Firth, J., Schuch, F. B., et al. 2017, 'Sedentary behavior and physical activity levels in people with schizophrenia, bipolar disorder and major depressive disorder: a global systematic review and meta-analysis', *World Psychiatry*, vol. 16, no. 3, pp. 308–315.

Vieta, E., Berk, M., Schulze, T. G., et al. 2018, 'Bipolar disorders', *Nat.Rev.Dis.Primers.*, vol. 4, p. 18008.

Vieta, E., Torrent, C., & Martínez-Arán, A. 2014, *Functional Remediation for Bipolar Disorder*. Cambridge: Cambridge University Press.

Vos, T., Flaxman, A. D., Naghavi, M., et al. 2012, 'Years lived with disability (YLDs) for 1160 sequelae of 289 diseases and injuries 1990–2010: a systematic analysis for the Global Burden of Disease Study 2010', *Lancet*, vol. 380, no. 9859, pp. 2163–2196.

Williams, J. M., Alatiq, Y., Crane, C., et al. 2008, 'Mindfulness-based Cognitive Therapy (MBCT) in bipolar disorder: preliminary evaluation of immediate effects on between-episode functioning', *J.Affect. Disord.*, vol. 107, no. 1–3, pp. 275–279.

Wykes, T., & Spaulding, W. D. 2011, 'Thinking about the future cognitive remediation therapy – what works and could we do better?', *Schizophr.Bull.*, vol. 37, Suppl. 2, pp. S80–S90.

Yatham, L. N., Kennedy, S. H., Parikh, S. V., et al. 2018, 'Canadian Network for Mood and Anxiety Treatments (CANMAT) and International Society for Bipolar Disorders (ISBD) 2018 guidelines for the management of patients with bipolar disorder', *Bipolar. Disord.*, vol. 20, no. 2, pp. 97–170.

Zaretsky, A., Lancee, W., Miller, C., Harris, A., & Parikh, S. V. 2008, 'Is cognitive-behavioural therapy more effective than psychoeducation in bipolar disorder?', *Can.J.Psychiatry*, vol. 53, no. 7, pp. 441–448.

Index

abstraction, selective 92
acceptance
  in mindfulness 11, 43, 45,
    89–90, 92
  in psychoeducation 17, 20,
    25, 28, 82, 83
acetylcholine 3, 65, 82
acronyms 100
action plan 22, 29, 69–70
active listening 108
activity levels, increased 66–67
acute episodes, interventions in
  5, 9–10
addictive disorders 21–22, 37, 79
aggression 106
alarms, use of 99
alcohol 22, 37, 79
allowing 41, 89–90
alprazolam 80
alternative therapies 72
amygdala 2, 52
anchorage 87–88
anticonvulsants 71
antidepressants 5, 35, 71, 77, 80
antipsychotics 5, 71, 84
anxiety
  anxiolytics 38, 71
  emotional hunger 35
  mindfulness use 11, 40
  nicotine withdrawal 80
appetite, changes in 35
arbitrary inference 92
aripiprazole 71
asenapine 71
assertiveness 39, 59, 106–109
assessment 32, 44
association 99
attachment 89
attendance 110
attention
  attention regulation 43
  cognitive and functional
    remediation 58, 95–96
  daily activities and 51
  deficits in bipolar disorder
    10, 50, 94
  eating 77, 88
  in mindfulness 11, 41–48,
    86–89, 90

automatic pilot, awareness
    versus 84–88
autonomy 59, 83
aversion 89
avoidance 30, 89–90
awareness
  body 43, 47–48, 90
  emotional 93
  in mindfulness 84–88, 93
  psychoeducation 19–20

Barcelona Bipolar and
    Depressive Disorders Unit
    ix, 15, 27–30, 55–60
behaviour
  aggressive 106
  assertive 39, 59, 106–109
  emotions and 93
  inhibition of 101, 102
  passive 106
  requesting change in 108
beliefs
  diagnosis 17
  erroneous 17, 20, 29, 58, 62, 66
  family 25, 27–28, 29
  stress management and 38
benzodiazepines 38, 71, 80
binge eating 77
biological basis (of bipolar
    disorder) 2–3
  integrative approach session
    material 64, 65, 82
biological rhythms 32–33
bipolar disorders
  bipolar I disorder 2
  bipolar II disorder 2
  introduction to 1–5
blame 83, 84
body awareness 43, 47–48, 90
body mass index (BMI) 34
brain
  frontal lobes 101
  limbic system 2, 52, 64
brainstorming 105
breathing
  controlled/diaphragmatic 81
  in mindfulness 45, 47,
    87–88, 89
bupropion 71, 80

caffeine 22, 37, 80
calendar, use of 99
cannabis 22, 79
carbamazepine 71, 84
carbohydrates 75
caregivers See also family
  family intervention 8–9
  positive role aspects 25
  self-care 84
cariprazine 71
catastrophism 91
categorisation 100
causes (of bipolar disorder) 2–3
  integrative approach session
    material 64–66, 82
change
  adaptation to 50, 59
  requesting behavioural 108
chunking 99
circadian rhythm 9, 32–33
  interpersonal and social
    rhythm therapy
    (IPSRT) 9–10
citalopram 71
classification, of bipolar
    disorders 2
clinical course 20
  factors influencing 3–4
clinical staging 4
clozapine 71
cocaine 80
coffee 22, 37, 80
cognition
  deficits in See cognitive
    deficits/impairment
  social 51–52
  stress management and 38
cognitive and functional
    enhancement/remediation
    10–11
cognitive remediation 10,
    50–55
functional remediation
    10–11, 50, 56–59
integrative approach module
    overview 60
integrative approach session
    material (attention and
    memory) 94–100

integrative approach session
material (executive
functions) 101–104
cognitive approach, working
with thoughts 91–92
cognitive-behavioural therapy
(CBT) 7
combined
psychoeducation 7
healthy lifestyle
promotion 32
research studies 7
cognitive deficits/impairment
50–52, 94–95
daily functioning
consequences 95
factors affecting conditions
52–53
prevention or improvement
approaches 54–55
psychosocial functioning
and 10
relapse frequency and 4
therapeutic target 4, 10, 54
cognitive flexibility 101
Cognitive Remediation Experts
Workshop 55
cognitive reserve 53, 95
enhancement of 54
communication rules, group
62, 110
communication skills training
attentional capacity 96
family 9, 26, 29–30
integrative approach session
material 106–109
stress management 39, 59
comorbidity 4, 37, 53, 61
concentration 50
confidentiality 110
conflict 83
avoidance of 30
conscious eating 35
conversation skills 109
coping strategies, planning
family 29
cortisol 53
co-therapist 62
criticism 9, 25, 26, 28, 83, 84
facing 109
self-criticism 41
curiosity 45, 48, 86

decision making 69, 105
delegation 102
denial 17, 25, 28, 41, 83

depression 1–2
action plan 70
acute phases 5
differences between unipolar
and bipolar 5
eating patterns 35
family intervention 9
integrative approach session
material 64, 67–68, 70
interpersonal and social
rhythm therapy (IPSRT) 10
mindfulness use 11, 40
nutrition and risk of 31
physical exercise and 79
psychoeducation 8
psychological interventions
in acute phase 5
designer drugs 80
desvenlafaxine 71
diagnosis 1
adjustment to 17
early 1, 4–5
Diagnostic and Statistical
Manual of Mental
Disorders (DSM) 1
dialectical behaviour therapy
(DBT) 12
diary, use of 98, 99
diazepam 80
dichotomous reasoning 92
diet See also nutrition
low sodium 71, 77
monoamine oxidase
inhibitors (MAOIs) 77
direct experience 86
Disability Adjusted Life Years
(DALY) 31
distractions 101, 104, 110
diuretics 71
dopamine 2, 65, 82
drug abuse 21, 37, 79–80
dual pathology 37
duloxetine 71

early detection (new episode)
22, 28, 66–70
eating See also diet; nutrition
conscious 35
mindful 88
overeating 35
economic decisions 70
education
cognitive reserve
enhancement 53
functional remediation
57–58

impact of disorder
education 17
psychoeducation See
psychoeducation
Eisenhower matrix 104
electroconvulsive therapy
(ECT) 71
emergency plan 22, 29, 69–70
emotions 93
bodily component of 90
diagnosis 17
emotional hunger 35
emotional reasoning 92
emotional regulation 11, 39,
44, 93
high expressed emotion 9,
25–26
in mindfulness See
mindfulness
social cognition and 52
transitory nature of 43
empathy 52
employment 33, 54, 74
energy drinks 37, 80
energy levels
increased 66–67
nutrition and 74–75
environmental factors
conscious eating and
environmental control
34
family psychoeducation
82–83
integrative approach session
material 65–66
sleep-related 73
triggers 2
vulnerability and 18, 19
escitalopram 71
euphoria 33
euthymia
cognitive deficits in 10
duration of 3
psychoeducation timing
27
evaluation 111
executive functions
cognitive and functional
enhancement/remediation
59, 95, 101–104
daily activities and 51
deficits in bipolar disorder
10, 50
integrative approach session
material 95, 101–104
exercise See physical exercise

exercises
  cognitive and functional
    enhancement/remediation
    100, 103
  mindfulness 88, 89, 91, 94
expectations, adjustment of
  84
experience, direct 86
exposure 44
expressed emotion 9, 25–26
eye movement desensitisation
  and reprocessing
  (EMDR) 12

family See also caregivers
  beliefs 25, 27–28, 29
  family burden 9, 24–26
  family intervention in
    bipolar disorder 8
  family studies 3
  functional remediation 58
  integrative approach session
    material 82–84
  psychoeducation 8–9, 17–18,
    24–30, 82–84
  stress/stress management
    24–26, 29–30
fats, healthy 76
feelings, expression of 108
flexibility 102
  cognitive 101
fluoxetine 71
fluvoxamine 71
frontal lobes, brain 101
functional remediation 50 See
  also cognitive and
    functional enhancement/
    remediation
  implementation formats 56
  introduction to 55–56
  timing of interventions 56

GABA 3
General Adaptation Model 38
genetics
  factors in bipolar disorder 2,
    3, 65
  family psychoeducation 82
  integrative approach session
    material 65
glutamate 3
group therapy
  family interventions 26
  functional remediation
    11, 56
  integrative approach 61–63

psychoeducation 8, 18–19, 26
rules 62, 110
guilt 28, 41, 92

habits, regularity of 22–23,
  73–81
hallucinogens 80
haloperidol 71
healthy lifestyle promotion
  importance of 4, 31–32
  integrative approach module
    overview 39
  integrative approach session
    material 73–81
  programme characteristics
    32–39
  research studies 32
high expressed emotion 9, 25–26
hippocampus 2, 52, 53
homework 63, 91, 94
hormonal factors 3, 53, 65, 82
hospitalisation, reduction in 8, 9
hostility 9
hydration 76
hypercortisolaemia 53
hyperphagia 35
hypersomnia 33, 70, 74
hypervigilance 25–26, 28, 83
hypnotics 38, 71
hypomania 1–2
  action plan 69–70
  antidepressant risk 71
  eating patterns 35
  integrative approach session
    material 64, 67, 68, 69–70
  physical exercise reduction
    36, 79
  sleep disturbance and 33
hypothalamus 2

imagery, visual 100
impulsivity, control of 102
inference, arbitrary 92
insomnia 71, 74
instructions, self-instructions
  96, 101
integrative approach
  cognitive and functional
    enhancement module
    overview 60
  healthy lifestyle promotion
    module overview 39
  mindfulness module
    overview 49
  participant satisfaction
    survey 111

psychoeducational module
  overview 30
  reasons for 15
  session material See
    integrative approach
    (session material)
  session organisation 61–62
  summary of content 63
  target group 61
  therapist's role 62–63
integrative approach (session
  material)
  Assertiveness and
    Communication Skills
    106–109
  Bipolar Disorder – Causes
    and Triggers 64–66
  Cognitive and Functional
    Enhancement – Attention
    and Memory 94–100
  Cognitive and Functional
    Enhancement – Executive
    Functions 101–104
  Mindfulness I – Automatic
    Pilot Versus Awareness
    84–88
  Mindfulness II – Habits of
    The Mind and
    The Importance of
    The Body 88–90
  Mindfulness III – Thoughts
    and Emotions 91–93
  Problem Solving 104–106
  Psychoeducation Directed to
    Family Members 82–84
  Regularity of Habits and
    Healthy Lifestyle 73–81
  Symptoms of Bipolar
    Disorder – Early Detection
    of Warning Signs and
    Early Action 66–70
  Treatment of Bipolar
    Disorder and Therapeutic
    Adherence 70–73
intelligence quotient (IQ)
  53
intention 43
interaction, social 78
interferences, controlling 101,
  104, 110
International Classification of
  Diseases (ICD) 1
Internet-supported
  psychological
  interventions 11–12,
  23–24, 101

interpersonal and social
  rhythm therapy
  (IPSRT) 9–10
interpretation 92
isolation, social 54

Jacobson's progressive muscle
  relaxation 81
judgements, hasty 92

kindness 86

labelling 92
lamotrigine 71, 84
letting go 90, 92
library metaphor 96–97
life expectancy 31
lifestyle interventions
  healthy lifestyle promotion
    See healthy lifestyle
    promotion
  research studies 13
limbic system 2, 52, 64
list making 99
listening skills 59, 96, 108
lithaemias 84
lithium 35, 70–71, 77, 83, 84
lorazepam 80
loss, sense of 17
lurasidone 71

magnification, of the
  negative 92
maintenance treatment 5,
  70, 83
mania 1–2
  action plan 69–70
  antidepressant risk 71
  antimanic drugs 71
  eating patterns 35
  integrative approach session
    material 64, 66–67, 68,
    69–70
  physical exercise reduction
    36, 79
  psychoeducation 8
  sleep disturbance and 33
manic-depressive syndrome 1
medication adherence See
  treatment adherence
medication misuse 80
memory
  cognitive and functional
    remediation 10, 11, 58–59,
    96–101
  daily activities and 51

deficits in bipolar disorder
  10, 50, 52, 94
mental filter 92
metacognitive training 12
metaphors
  library metaphor for
    memory 96–97
  mindfulness 45–46
method of the 3 readings 96
mind reading 92
mindfulness
  assessment instruments 44
  benefits of 87
  components of 43–44
  different practice types
    44–46
  emotional regulation 39
  exercises 88, 89, 91, 94
  importance of practice 46–48
  integrative approach
    mindfulness session
    I material (Automatic
    Pilot versus Awareness)
    84–88
  integrative approach
    mindfulness session II
    material (Habits of the
    Mind and The Importance
    of The Body) 88–90
  integrative approach
    mindfulness session III
    material – Thoughts and
    Emotions 91–93
  integrative approach session
    material (Regularity of
    Habits) 73–81
  intervention types 42–43
  introduction to 40–42
  mindfulness-based cognitive
    therapy (MBCT) 11, 42–43
  mindfulness-based stress
    reduction (MBSR) 11, 42
  reasons for integrative
    approach inclusion
    48–49
  relaxation differentiation 85
  research studies 48
mirtazapine 71
mixed symptoms 2, 68
mnemonic rules 99–100
mobile-based interventions
  11–12, 23–24, 101
MONARCA (MONitoring,
  treatment and pRediCtion
  of bipolAr Disorder
  Episodes) 24

monoamine oxidase inhibitors
  (MAOIs) 35, 77
mood stabilisers 5, 35,
  70–71, 83
mood states See also specific
  mood states
  episode types in bipolar
    disorder 64
  family psychoeducation 82
mortality rates 4, 31
motivation 32, 78
  cannabis-related
    amotivational
    syndrome 79
muscle relaxation 81
myths 17, 20, 29, 58, 62, 66

names, remembering 100
negative feelings, expression
  of 108
negative thoughts 90
neurocognitive training 10 See
  also cognitive and
  functional enhancement/
  remediation
neuroendocrine system 3
neurotransmitters 2, 65, 82
nicotine replacement therapy
  37, 80
noradrenaline 2, 65, 82
notes, as reminders 99
nutrition See also diet; eating
  benefits of good dietary
    habits 31
  food patterns in bipolar
    disorders 31
  healthy lifestyle promotion
    33–36, 74–77
  integrative approach session
    material 74–77
  research studies 13
  sleep patterns and 73

obesity 32, 33
observation, in mindfulness
  86–87, 90, 92–93
olanzapine 71, 84
omega-3 fatty acids 77
onset, of bipolar disorder 1,
  64
openness 45, 48
organisational skills 50,
  101–104 See also planning
outcomes 15
overeating 35
overgeneralisation 92

overprotection 25–26, 28, 83, 84
oxcarbazepine 71

pain
  observation of 90
  resistance/acceptance of 89–90
paliperidone 71
paroxetine 71
participation 110
passivity 106
patience 84
patterns, detection of 20
perception 81, 93
personalisation 92
personality 65
perspective, change in 44
pharmacological treatments
    See also specific drugs/drug types
  adherence to See treatment adherence
  dietary considerations 35
  family psychoeducation 83–84
  importance of adjunctive psychological treatments 6–7
  integrative approach session material 70–71, 83–84
  maintenance 5, 70, 83
  medication misuse 80
  overview 4–5
  side effects See side effects
physical exercise
  benefits of 31
  healthy lifestyle promotion 36–37, 77–79
  integrative approach session material 77–79
  research studies 13
  sleep patterns and 73
pill boxes 99
planning
  cognitive and functional enhancement/remediation 59, 101–104
  difficulties in bipolar disorder 50
  emergency 22, 29, 69
  family coping strategies 82–83
  integrative approach session material 101–104, 106
  meal 76

physical exercise 78
problem solving 106
stress prevention 81
positive feelings 108
postpartum period 3, 65
practice See also exercises
  of mindfulness 86–88
pregnancy 21
prevalence
  of bipolar disorder 1, 64
  of cognitive impairment 50
prioritisation 102–104
problem solving
  cognitive and functional remediation 10, 39, 59
  family 26, 30
  integrative approach session material 39, 59, 104–106
  psychoeducation 26, 30
  research studies 9
processing speed 10, 51
pro-cognitive drugs 54
prodromes 22, 28, 68–70
prognosis 4
protective factors 20, 66
proteins 75
psychoeducation 8
  aspects of 18, 26
  awareness 19–20
  cognitive impairment therapy 54
  combined cognitive-behavioural therapy (CBT) 7
  contents of 19, 27–30
  family 9, 17–18, 24–30, 82–84
  functional remediation and 11
  implementation formats 18–19, 26
  integrative approach overview 30
  patient 17–24
  research studies 8, 19
  timing of 19, 27
psychological treatments See also specific treatments
  duration of sessions 15
  evidence for common approaches 7–10
  importance of 6–7
  integrative approach session material 72, 84
  new approaches 10–13
  outcomes 15

overview 5
  reasons for integrative approach 15
  targets of 6
psychosocial functioning See also cognitive and functional enhancement/remediation
  cognitive deficits and 10, 54
  relapse frequency and 4
  treatment target 4
punctuality 110

quetiapine 10, 71, 84

rapid-cycling 71
reading 96
reappraisal 44
record sheet, activity planning 102
reflective listening 96
refusal, of requests 108
relapse
  early detection of 22, 28
  prevention of 7–10, 19
  prognosis and frequency of 4
relaxation
  mindfulness differentiation 41, 85
  techniques 81, 84
repetition, technique of 100
request refusal 108
research studies
  cognitive-behavioural therapy (CBT) 7
  family intervention 8–9
  family studies 3
  healthy lifestyle promotion 32
  interpersonal and social rhythm therapy (IPSRT) 9–10
  mindfulness 48
  new psychological treatments 10–13
  psychoeducation 8, 19
  twin studies 3
residual symptoms 1, 3
resistance 41, 46, 89–90
respect 106–107, 110
rhythm/rhyming 100
rights, of the individual 106–107
risperidone 71
rules, group format 62, 63, 110

satisfaction, with intervention 111
selective abstraction 92
self-care, caregiver's 84
self-criticism 41
self-instructions 96, 101
Self-Monitoring and Psychoeducation in Bipolar Patients with a Smartphone application (SIMPLe) 23–24
serotonin 2, 65, 82
sertraline 71
shame 20
side effects
    antidepressants 71
    antipsychotics 71
    cognitive impairment 53, 54
    electroconvulsive therapy (ECT) 71
    lithium 70
    treatment adherence and 72
    weight gain 35, 77
SIMPLe 23–24
sleep
    factors affecting cognition 53
    healthy lifestyle promotion characteristics 32–33
    hypersomnia 33, 70, 74
    insomnia 71, 74
    integrative approach session material 73–74
    new episode action plan 69, 70
    physical exercise timing 36, 79
    sleep hygiene guidelines 73–74
    stimulant substances and 37, 80
Smartbands 78
smoking/smoking cessation 37, 80
social cognition 51–52
social interaction 78
social isolation 54
sodium levels 71, 77
stigma 17, 20, 62
stimulant substances 22, 37, 80
story-telling 100
stress
    as a trigger 4, 9, 80
    definition of 38
    emotional hunger 35
    family 9, 24–26

management of See stress management
    prevention of 81
    response to 80
    stress-vulnerability model 19
stress management
    family psychoeducation 24–26, 29–30
    functional remediation 59
    importance in integrative approach 38–39
    integrative approach session material 80–81
    mindfulness overview 40
    mindfulness-based stress reduction (MBSR) 11, 42
    patient psychoeducation 22–23
    sleep patterns 33
    substance abuse
    healthy lifestyle promotion 37–38
    integrative approach session material 79
    prevalence of 4
    psychoeducation 21–22
suffering, accepting/ allowing 90
suicide risk 4
susceptibility threshold model 3
symbolic reminders 99
symptoms
    communication and 107
    family understanding of 28
    integrative approach session material 66–70
    mixed 2, 68
    overview of 1–2
    problem solving and 104
    residual 1, 3

targets, treatment 4, 10, 54
technology
    cognitive and functional remediation 98, 101
    controlling disturbance by 104
    Internet-supported psychological interventions 11–12, 23–24, 101
    physical exercise monitoring 78
    psychoeducation 23–24
    sleep-pattern recording 33

terminology 1
thalamus 2
theory of mind 52
therapists, role of 62–63
thoughts 91–93
    in mindfulness See mindfulness
    negative 86, 90
    thinking versus experiencing 43
    transitory nature of 43
thyroid hormones 3, 65, 82
time management 59, 101, 102–104
time thieves 104
timing, of interventions 19, 27, 56
tobacco 37, 80
tolerance 84
traumatic events 12
trazodone 71
treatment See also specific treatments
    impact of 66
    overview of 4–5
    targets 4, 10, 54
treatment adherence
    clinical course and 3
    cognitive and functional remediation 99
    family psychoeducation 29, 83–84
    integrative approach session material 72, 83–84
    patient psychoeducation 20–21
    psychological therapy impact 6
    reasons for poor 72
triggers
    circadian rhythm instability 9
    disrupted routines 9
    integrative approach session material 64–66
    sleep-related 9, 33
    stress 4, 9, 80
    substance abuse 37
twin studies 3

valproate 71, 84
varinicline 80
vegetables 75
venlafaxine 71
visual imagery 100
visual learning 10

vortioxetine 71
vulnerability, environmental factors and 18, 19

walking 79
water intake 76

web-based interventions 11–12, 23–24, 101
weight gain 33, 35, 77
well-being 38, 80

enhancement in integrative approach 38–39
integrative approach session material 80–81

ziprasidone 71